Speech Therapy

Effective Speech Therapy Strategies for Children

(Helpful Games and Therapy Ideas for Parents to Try at Home)

Eduardo Bush

Published By **Darby Connor**

Eduardo Bush

All Rights Reserved

Speech Therapy: Effective Speech Therapy Strategies for Children (Helpful Games and Therapy Ideas for Parents to Try at Home)

ISBN 978-1-77485-581-2

No part of this guidebook shall be reproduced in any form without permission in writing from the publisher except in the case of brief quotations embodied in critical articles or reviews.

Legal & Disclaimer

The information contained in this ebook is not designed to replace or take the place of any form of medicine or professional medical advice. The information in this ebook has been provided for educational & entertainment purposes only.

The information contained in this book has been compiled from sources deemed reliable, and it is accurate to the best of the Author's knowledge; however, the Author cannot guarantee its accuracy and validity and cannot be held liable for any errors or omissions. Changes are periodically made to this book. You must consult your doctor or get professional medical advice before using any of the suggested remedies, techniques, or information in this book.

Upon using the information contained in this book, you agree to hold harmless the Author from and against any damages, costs, and expenses, including any legal fees potentially resulting from the application of any of the information provided by this guide. This disclaimer applies to any damages or injury caused by the use and application, whether directly or indirectly, of any advice or information presented, whether for breach of contract, tort, negligence, personal injury, criminal intent, or under any other cause of action.

You agree to accept all risks of using the information presented inside this book. You need to consult a professional medical practitioner in order to ensure you are both able and healthy enough to participate in this program.

Table Of Contents

Introduction 1

Chapter 1: The Basics 2

Chapter 2: What Is Listening Skills? 10

Chapter 3: Let's Get Specific! 18

Chapter 4: Grade Level-Listening Skills... 38

Chapter 5: Strategies And Activities 44

Chapter 6: Speech And Language Development 79

Chapter 7: The Language Delays And Disorders 92

Chapter 8: Speech Sound Delays And Disorders 101

Chapter 9: The Conditions That Are Influenced By Social Conditions 110

Chapter 10: Down Syndrome 115

Chapter 11: Interaction Between A Child And A Parent 120

Chapter 12: Language As Well As Makaton To Speech And Language Development 127

Chapter 13: The Treatments You Can Try At Home.. 133

Chapter 14: The Understanding Of Articulation And Phonological Disorder 174

Conclusion 181

Introduction

Parents watching your child struggle to speak clearly is painful. It's difficult to watch your child struggle to communicate with simple speech, struggling to convey the hunger he feels or articulate his feelings when he's upset or angry. A child's inability to communicate what he desires can be difficult for both the child and the parent.

It is essential to get your child's illness diagnosed at the earliest possible time and to begin treatment as soon as possible. What if I told you that there's something you could do to help also?

The book contains a variety of speech therapy exercises parents can do with their children who suffer from articulation or phonological disorders in order to develop their child's language. It begins by helping you the condition of your child and the root cause of the disorder. After you've pinpointed the root of the problem, treatment and therapy can be initiated. The exercises in this book have been designed to be enjoyable and engaging in order to keep your child excited and wanting to take part.

Chapter 1: The Basics

Every subject and every subject each and every activity and every profession has its own vocabulary. I believe I'm intelligent until I listen to the husband of my son and his friend from fishing discussing fishing. At that point, I don't know what they're discussing.

It's like speaking in a different language, and it is, at the very least, to my eyes.

Communication is not any different. Therefore, before we can begin to tackle the details of developing your child's listening skills it is necessary to have an understanding of the basics of the terms and concepts regarding speaking and language. Let's begin with the most obvious.

What is an audiologist?

A speech therapist, also known as a speech pathologist is someone who has been specially trained to diagnose and treat disorders of communication. When I started my career, I was referred to as the speech therapist. Later I was a speech pathologist. When I retired, I was an slp. Three terms can be used to refer to the same job.

Speech pathologists may work in private or in clinics that specialize in speech therapy and in public schools. Every public school in the country is required to offer speech therapy to children with disabilities in communication. If you suspect that your child may have an issue with communication contact the community school's district would be a great first step.

Communication is what it's all about.

My understanding of communications is that a person communicates the message to a listener and the recipient is able to receive the message exactly as it was intended to be received.

Three elements are included in this description: sender of the message, the recipient of the message, and finally the message that is intended to be sent.

The word that is most important is meant.

The speaker can deliver the message and the audience might receive the message however if the message isn't comprehended as intended, then communication did not occur. It's more likely to be an interruption in communication. A bad situation in the majority of circumstances. To be able to communicate the person listening must be able to comprehend the message the speaker has sent.

Language and communication are not the same thing, even though many believe that.

What is a language?

The definition of language is a system of undefined symbols that have rules utilized to convey thoughts, ideas and emotions. What? To gain a better understanding of what this means , let's take a look in pieces.

Language is a set of random symbols. This is a complex method of saying that words are symbolic, not actually objects. You've probably heard this, but you may have not thought of it this way prior to.

This is the case for all words. They represent the object. Chair is not actually a chair. It was decided long ago that the item would be referred to as a chair. It could have as easily been referred to as a couch. A dog could just as easily been referred to as cat.

This is what's meant by random symbols.

The only time a set of people who speak a language be able to agree on the term DOG to mean the animal with four legs , an animal tail, as well as barks, that the word can take the meaning. It is possible that the word "cat" could could have been used to refer to the dog and CAT could be the name that we use to describe the animal we recognize as the dog.

I hope this makes sense.

Language is a set of random symbols that have rules.

The rules enable people to write unlimited sentences that people who speak the same language are able to comprehend. If a person doesn't understand or apply the rules correctly the possibility of a breakdown in communication could occur.

Language is a set of random symbols and rules used to convey thoughts, ideas and emotions.

Language is a tool that we utilize for a myriad of uses, like educating or seeking information or to communicate, as well as to share ideas or thoughts. Language is used to accomplish many purposes including those that are listed above.

Let's examine the definition a second time. The language is a set that consists of symbols and rules utilized to convey thoughts, ideas and feelings.

It will make sense right now.

In order to make things confusing further The language skills are classified in various ways. One of the most commonly used is to classify them into expressive and receptive communication skills.

Receptive language skills indicate that we are able to comprehend the language spoken by others. Expression skills are capabilities we employ to express our thoughts and thoughts.

They can then be broken down further into distinct components. These components aid us in testing our language proficiency, but we don't usually think about the components as we talk since they all play a role to create what we consider to be the language.

These components include:

Pragmatic

Phonology

Semantics

Morphology

Syntax

Pragmatics

Pragmatics is the part of language that addresses the question: Why do we communicate? Communication can be a result of different reasons, but we require a reason. To be a proficient user of language your child should be able to communicate in a variety of ways with various people in various situations.

Phonology

Phonology is the branch of linguistics which is concerned with the phonetic system of the language. Also, it is how we talk or talk.

Phonology goes beyond the actual creation of speech sounds. It is the set of rules that govern the way we use the language's sound system. For instance In English we don't use an NG sounds at the start of words but in other languages, it is a common sound combination.

Semantics

Semantics is the part of language that handles meaning, also known as vocabulary. The development of vocabulary is essential for becoming an effective user of language.

Morphology

Morphology is a part of language which deals with the rules of forming acceptable words. It addresses such issues as suffixes, prefixes, plurals, singulars as well as verb tenses.

English is particularly difficult in this field. As an example, a house is two houses while mouse turns into 2 mice. Children who suffer from expressive language disorders typically struggle dealing with the morphology of English.

Syntax

Syntax is the process of creating sentences that are acceptable in the language. Syntax is about the order of words. When you combine syntax and Morphology, you've got the grammar of the language. And , yes, I believe the importance of grammar.

As you can observe it is evident that the study of language and communication is a complicated topic. There's been a number of books published about the subject of language and its elements as innumerable research studies that were conducted in the past, and being conducted today.

At this point, you may be frightened. You may be thinking you'll never be able to assist your child develop their speech and language skills , and more specifically, their listening abilities.

Stop! !

Yes, the subject of language and communication is complex, but making your child's speech skills better isn't as hard as you may believe. Like I've said before parents have always been the most effective and first teachers of language. Yes, you can do it!

So , take a deep breathe and read.

Chapter 2: What Is Listening Skills?

Listening is the foundation for learning a language and for learning to communicate with other people. If you are unable to comprehend the message according to the intention and you don't understand the message, then communication hasn't been achieved.

Listening and hearing are not the identical. Listening is the bodily process of hearing the sounds. Listening means being able identify the meaning of those sounds. It is possible to be a perfect listener and be unable to listen.

Listening skills are known by a myriad of names. Processing of language, auditory or auditory comprehension, receptive language , and listening abilities, call it whatever you prefer They all mean the identical things. It is the process of learning to comprehend spoken language. Skills in listening are essential to success in the classroom and throughout life.

Language is used for a myriad of purposes, however, we accomplish this in just four ways.

We listen.

We talk.

We read.

We write.

Whatever the reason you choose to use language or what you intend to accomplish, these are the methods to achieve it. Then we build those abilities in exactly the same sequence that I described them in. The first step is listening, followed by speaking, reading, and finally , writing.

As you can see , listening is the first step, which is why it's essential to begin communicating with your children from the moment they are born and keep talking. Listening is the very first step towards becoming a fluent speaker. Therefore, listening skills impact all other aspects that develop language.

A speech and language therapist I didn't feel like there was enough time available to spend alongside my pupils. There were so many demands and I was able to fill in the gaps with so little time. As I gained experience I began to realize the importance of developing my listening abilities.

If I could only choose one language area I could focus on for a child who is struggling at school I would recommend enhancing listening skills. A good listening ability is the most important factor in developing good communication skills and succeeding in the academic environment.

The ability to listen better can help improve other aspects of language.

In order for children to succeed at school, they should be ready to tackle all of the activities required. The majority of these activities depend heavily on the ability to communicate. What is the best way to teach?

In the majority of cases the two of them talk while the child listens, but then the roles reverse, and your child is talking while the teacher is listening. Therefore, in order to ensure that your child's success at school, you must aid them in reaching their full capabilities by helping improve their communication and language abilities, particularly listening skills. It starts with the ability to comprehend what they hear.

Based on my personal experience I've observed that the lack of listening skills is one of the primary reason why children struggle to achieve success at school. If you are able to improve your listening skills, that can make a huge difference in making them more successful in school.

Does your child have the ability to be an excellent listener? Here are some of the questions that can assist you in answering this question.

Is your child a good LISTNER?

1. Does your child glance at you or others when they speak?

2. Does your child have difficulty understanding body language or facial expressions?

3. Do you need to contact your child multiple times before they finally respond to you?

4. Does your child often say "huh" or "what" often?

5. Do your children often need to be reminded of questions, details or instructions?

6. Does your child display you were misunderstood by his your actions or words?

7. Do your children have trouble recalling stories, songs and nursery rhymes?

8. Does your child's focus shift when you talk to them for longer than a couple of minutes?

9. Do you know if your child has trouble recalling people's names?

10. Do your children have trouble understanding new words or learning new information?

11. Do you have a child who has trouble understanding the meanings of new terms?

12. Do your children have difficulty comprehending new concepts?

13. Does your child have trouble understanding basic directions?

14. Do your children have trouble understanding 2 and 3 step directions, or more complex ones?

15. Do you have to repeat the directions 3 or 2 or four times before they understand it?

16. Do your children have trouble identifying with words that sound similar?

17. Does your child get the humor and jokes of your child?

18. Do you have a child who is easily distracted?

19. Are your children having difficulties in school, specifically when it comes to writing or reading?

20. Did your child's teacher inform the parent that your child is having difficulties paying attention at the classroom?

The answers to these questions will provide you with an idea of the need for your child to develop their listening skills. If you haven't yet done this then you must determine if they suffer from hearing impairment. This can be done by asking for an audiogram at your school or with an accredited auditory specialist.

My experience has been that improving the processing of language will improve the overall language skills of the majority of children. It helps improve their syntax and vocabulary and also improves their academic performance within the school environment.

As children develop into better at processing language as they develop, they start to see patterns in their the language and start to utilize the patterns on a regular basis in their expressive language abilities.

As I mentioned earlier, the fundamental foundation for learning in many classes is when the instructor speaks and students are able to listen. The same is true in a classroom for deaf students, except that the language may be both visual and auditory. Children who are deaf or hard of hearing must be able to comprehend the language, whether they're seeing or hearing it.

This is why I spent a large amount during their time with therapy enhancing their listening abilities or processing of language. Every time as their listening abilities improved, I observed an improvement in their all-language skills, both expressive and expressive.

What happens when a student struggles to process spoken language? He is unable to learn and comprehending the new information that is being presented. Naturally, he is unable to catch up. He becomes angry and frustrated as he's accused of not being a good person even though he is aware that he's trying. At some point, he stops trying since it isn't helping anyway.

He is more passive an observer rather than actively. Like Simon (1985a) observed, an active listener has the ability to discern the absence of information or unclear. This gives students to ask questions and clarify the meaning of the information.

Students are more likely to fully engage in the learning process or in the process of communication if they are able to listen effectively. A listener who is active makes an active part in the learning process and will increase the likelihood of the student to achieve success.

It is vital that students to improve their listening abilities to their fullest potential. As a result, students will become more effective speakers in all settings which includes home, school and at work. Understanding of language is the initial step towards becoming a proficient user of language.

However, even if your child is suffering from hearing impairment, enhancing their the ability to listen is essential for their development of language. Actually, it's even more important. Hearing levels isn't increased unless you use hearing aids or cochlear implant, however how much information that is processed and understood could increase whether hearing the language or using American Sign Language. If your child is suffering from hearing loss or is not, their listening skills are able to be improved.

Chapter 3: Let's Get Specific!

Once you've got an idea of the general concept of listening skills, or whatever term you like, let's get more specific. Listening skills can be classified or classified in a variety of ways. In this case we'll classify listening abilities into three distinct categories: pragmatic/social, phonetic; and language.

PRAGMATIC/SOCIAL SKILLS analyzes listening behavior from a communication viewpoint. Also, does your child display appropriate behaviors in listening to other people? These skills are essential to enable your child to be able to listen and learn in any setting (school or at home).

Eyes toward the speaker

Appropriate eye contact

Disconnects from distractions and focuses on the speaker

Responds promptly

Responds promptly to requests for assistance (Can I have some of your treats?)

Responds in a timely manner to indirect requests (That candy looks yummy as I'm hungry.)

Pragmatic social listening skills can be taught by modeling appropriate behaviour for your child, as well as talking about situations that arise. Children tend to improve in this aspect naturally as they get older.

PHONOLOGICAL LEVEL is concerned with our the phonology (sound) method. The most fundamental foundation is the sound of sounds that the form of words. In English we employ words to signify sounds. Certain letters may represent more sounds, and occasionally two or three letters can be joined to create other sounds.

Your child should have a solid understanding of the phonological system that is used in English and also the relationship between sounds and letters in order to be able to read and writing. Therefore, enhancing these skills is vital.

The ability of auditory discrimination to differentiate between sounds of two or more. This is crucial when hearing words that sound similar like WISTFUL-WISHFUL. If your child is struggling in this area, it may impact the development of vocabulary along with writing and reading.

Sound Blending is the capacity to detect sounds that are not distinct and then blend them together to form words. This is a crucial skill when your child starts to read. If you try to pronounce an word and end up with Ba-NaNa, but your brain doesn't interpret the word as bananas, you're likely cause it to be more difficult to read.

Auditory Segmenting is the capability to listen to a word and split it into smaller pieces of sound. It is the reverse of mixing sounds. It is also a vital aptitude to read. It is more challenging than sound mixing, but it is equally important.

Sound-symbol correspondence can be described as an elegant way of ensuring that your child can see a link between the sounds we speak and alphabets we study. This is essential to develop writing and reading skills.

Visual Sound-symbol corresponds to sound-symbol communication, but also the ability to read the written word and figure out the sounds the letters make.

The ability to recognize the sound position within words allows you to identify the place a sound appears within the word. Beginning--Middle--or End?

Rhyming is a crucial skill to develop as your child learns to write and read. Your child must be capable of recognizing and making up rhymes. Two levels are involved in rhyming which will aid your child with reading.

LINGUISTIC LEVEL is understanding connected speech. Does your child understand and interpret meaning across a range of situations? The Phonologic level concerns the sounds, as well as writing and reading, however the linguistic level is all about comprehending speech when it is used in social or academic contexts.

Auditory Memory refers to the ability to keep information that an individual hears. If someone isn't able to comprehend the information, they aren't able to recall it. This is also the case. If they don't recall the information, they'll have trouble understanding the information. It is usually measured using diverse tasks like following instructions, repeating words, numbers, or telling the story.

Auditory Perception refers to the ability to comprehend and receive sentences and words. That is, they can comprehend the meaning of what they hear. This ability impacts communication in various ways, such as vocabulary and concepts development, as well as social communication abilities.

Hearing Details Integration refers to the capacity to hear information and be capable of answering questions regarding it. This ability is essential to getting a good grade at the classroom.

The Auditory Vocal Association refers to the capability to discern relationships from it and respond to it verbally. Children who have difficulty in this area may struggle to complete basic sentences and solving puzzles and recognizing humor. They may not be able to answer the question asked.

We're all different which means we all learn differently. certain of us are visually-oriented, while others are auditory learners and a few lucky individuals are both auditory learners.

Should your child be not strong in the area of listening or auditory skills, there are many ways to improve the listening abilities of your child. It is first necessary to recognize the strengths and weaknesses of your child to give you an idea of the areas that are in need of improvement.

This checklist is not specifically geared towards a particular grade or age. It is a checklist of the fundamental skills children of school age need to be successful at school. Take this as a reference point. If your child is in the first or Kindergarten grades and is competent in certain skills. In the third or fourth grade they should be able to master all or a majority of the tasks.

DIRECTIONS. You can utilize a checkmark or "Y" for yes, and an N for no. Following the checklist, I've added specific exercises to help you determine if your child is equipped with these specific abilities.

Listening SKILLS Checklist

DATE OF SKILL the date:

SOCIAL/PRAGMATIC

Eyes the speaker.

Appropriate eye contact.

Attends the speaker.

Ignores distractions

Responds promptly.

Responds in a timely manner to any requests.

PHONOLOGICAL

Similar or different?

Sound Blending

Auditory Synthesis

Sound-symbol Correspondence

Recognizes the positions of sound in words

Recognizes rhymes

Creates rhymes

LINGUISTIC

Words are arranged in syntactic order

Follows 1 part directions

Follows 2 part directions

Follows 3 part directions

Follows intricate directions

Repeats 3-5 numbers

Repeats 3 numbers backwards

Repetition of short sentences

Nursery rhymes are repeated

Retells a short story

Incorporates auditory information with details

Answers questions appropriately

Paraphrases the latest information.

Instructions for Listening SKILLS A LISTENING RECORD

Social-Pragmatic Level The following are the basic behavior that a child must exhibit to demonstrate in order to be as a "good listener." These are the behaviors you need to observe frequently. Watch and then respond with yes or no.

Eyes the speaker.

Appropriate eye contact.

Attends a talk by speaker

Ignores distractions

Responds promptly

Responds promptly to any requests.

PHONOLOGICAL LEVEL The child should understand the phonetic system (sounds) in order to succeed in writing and reading.

Different or the same? Does your child know the difference between identical and different words? Keep your mouth shut and don't over-pronounce the words. If your child fails to speak more than 3words, this could be an indicator of a problem.

WORD LIST:

SIP-TIP

BALL-BALL

FILL-FELL

FISH-FIST

TEN-TENT

NEXT-NETS

WIND-WHEN

PEST-PAST

LIPS-LISP

SOP-SHOP

WISTFUL-WISHFUL

The ability to blend sounds can be described as the capacity to listen to distinct sounds and then blend them back together in the word. If you are assessing, select 10 words that your child will likely to recognize. If your child is missing more than three words, this could be a target.

WORD LIST:

BA-NA-NA

BI-CY-CLE

RE-MEM-BER

EL-E-PHANT

B-A-BY

ZE-BRA

L-E-MON

A-P-PLE

R-A-B-B-I-T

TA-B-LE

P-E-N-C-IL

M-O-N-K-EY

W-A-T-ER

W-I-N-T-ER

M-OU-SE

H-OU-SE

S-L-EE-P

S-I-NG

SEGMENTING AUDITORY It is the ability to listen to a word and then break it down into smaller parts of sounds. This is the opposite of mixing sounds. This is an essential capability to read. The following list of words can be used as a reference whether you have the skills. It is more challenging than mixing sounds. If your child is missing more than four times, it might be an opportunity to improve the.

SOUND-SYMBOL CORRESPONDENCE an elegant way to say that your child is aware of a link between the sounds we speak and the words we write. This is vital to reading comprehension.

It can be done in a variety of ways. Start by saying an alphabet sound. For example: buh. And then ask them to tell you the letter they used. Don't put them in sequence! Another option is to choose a letter, such as B. Then, ask them to explain the sounds it makes. Find any letter sounds your child isn't able to hear.

A B C D E F G H I J K L M N O P Q R S T U V W X Y Z

Visual SOUND-SYMBOL CORRESPONDENCE is the same as the one above but the child will identify a letter written in writing and can make the sound associated with the letter.

Buy or make an flash cards with the alphabet. Display the letters, and ask students to make the sound that each letter produces. Making the sound isn't the same as calling the letter. Your child should be aware of the sound every letter makes to be capable of "sound and spell" words.

A B C D E F G H I J K L M N O P Q R S T U V W X Y Z

Recognizing the sound's position in words The capability to recognize the location of a particular sound within the word. Beginning--Middle--or End?

Directions Instructions: Listen to the word , and determine which direction you think the S word is. Are you located in the middle, beginning or the end position?

1. House

2. sandy

3. Muscle

4. Pay attention

5. Save

6. Sorry

7. Mouse

8. mistake

9. Soon

10. scissors

If they are missing more than three skills, it could be an indication of a deficit in the skill.

Identifies the rhymes in a pair It is possible that your child does not be aware of what a rhyme is, so provide numerous examples prior to beginning. Tell me if the words rhyme, either yes or no. If they are missing more than three, try to improve this ability.

1. Dog/Frog

2. Bed/Red

3. Ten/Tin

4. Three/tree

5. Sit/Sing

6. Yes/No

7. Fun/Sun

8. Best/Rest

9. Maybe/Baby

10. Red/Blue

PRODUCES RHYMES: Pay attention and say an adjective in rhyme with the one I'm saying. If they don't have an rhyme for at least three of the words, then you need to work on this ability.

1. Log

2. Sat

3. Run

4. Had

5. Long

6. Cake

7. Sting

8. Boy

9. Not

10. Last

The LINGUISTIC LEVEL

Correct word order Listen to the words I'm saying, then turn them into an enunciation that is understandable. If they're unable to form at least five sentences that are good then they need to work on this skill.

SENTENCE LIST:

Dog See I see the (I can see I see the dog.)

Me and Danny and Danny (Danny had fun playing along together with me.)

Are lemons sour? (The lemons are so sour. Or, are the lemons sour?)

Claus fat is Santa (Santa Claus is fat.)

Bear brown, the brown bear (The bear had brown.)

Chocolate cake likes Mary. (Mary loves chocolate cakes.)

The comedy film was (The film was hilarious.)

Ringing phone (The phone is being rung.)

My sister and me laughing. was (My sister was laughing at me.)

Park where I lost my shoes (I have lost shoes in the park.).)

One-Part instructions: If they aren't able to accomplish the above, then focus on the ability.

STAND Up

Sit down

CUT your hands

STAY on the floor

PRESS your nose

Two-part instructions: If they fail to perform at least 4 or more of them, they should focus the skill.

STAND UP and TURN AROUND

Relax and touch your NOSE

CLAP YOUR HANDS and STAY on the floor

Toes should be touched, then you can jump up and down

START TURNING AROUND, THEN SET down

Three Part Instructions: If the person is unable to perform at least 3 (3) of the above, they should focus on the ability.

PICK A PEN UP, turn it around, and then sit down

PLACE THE PEN ON THE FLOR, JUMP, FINALLY SCRATCH your nose.

Sit down, pick up the pen, THROW IT IN your hands.

To touch your head CLAP YOUR HANDS, Then, sit down.

Turn around and then clasp your hands Then, JUMP UP and DOUBLE

Directions for Complex Make use of a piece of pencil and paper to complete this task. Repeat the instructions two or three times, but you must repeat the whole set of instructions. Don't break it down into distinct directions. If they fail to do at least one totally correct and one that is almost correct, then focus on this particular skill.

DRAW A LINE, PUT A CIRCLE OVER THE LINE AND A TRIANGLE UNDER THE LINE.DRAW A SQUARE, PUT 3 LINES IN IT, AND BIG CIRCLE AROUND IT.

Draw 3 circles in a Row, and then draw a line between the FIRST and LAST CIRCLES. PUT AN X in the MIDDLE CIRCLE.

Draw a triangle between two CIRCLES and PUT A line in the middle, then put a line underneath each of the CIRCLES.

Draw 5 squares in a row. Put a line under the MIDDLE SQUARE. PLACE AN X ON THE FIRST SQUARE.

NUMBER REPITITION For children who are five years old or over and is five or over, they should be able repeatedly repeat the entire list back. Don't repeat them all at once. Tell your child, "Please repeat back the numbers

I've given you. Pay attention because I'll only say them one time."

5-8-3

14-5-20

2-12-31

67-45-92

11-84-51

NUMBER REPITITION IN REVERSE When your kid is older than six years old, they should be able say all the numbers in reverse. Speak to them "I am going to repeat numbers and I would like you to do them backwards. If I were to say, 3-5 you'd say 5-3. Let me try one. Tell me 2-8. Listen carefully. I'll only repeat them one time."

8-2-7

6-3-4

10-5-9-1

8-12-4-16

17-5-2-8-4

SHORT sentence recitation If they aren't able to do at minimum 3 correctly, they should target the skill.

This dog's color is black.

It's raining outside.

I don't like mean dogs.

My sister is five years old.

Mark is a fan of going to school.

NURSERY RHYMES: Pick the one your kid is not familiar with. Repeat it several times and then let them practice it independently. If they are able to say it correctly, that's fine.

Jack and Jill

Humpty Dumpty

Hickory Dickory Dock

Retell a Story You can tell your child an interesting story they are not familiar with. Retell them the story. If they are able to recall the most important details in the right order, that's fine.

Little Red Riding Hood

Three Little Pigs

Jack and the Beanstalk

AUDITORY DETAILS INTERGRATION: Can your child listen to the information and later answer questions regarding the information they heard? They should be able answer at least two questions following listening to the brief paragraph.

John Robert and John Robert had brothers. John had been 13 when he was born, and Robert aged 10. The other day, John as well as Robert had a game of baseball. John was throwing his ball towards Robert but the ball was thrown too far. The ball instead hit the window of their garage.

1. What was the older brother?

2. What happened after the ball struck the window?

3. What do you think they should do?

COMPREHEND INFORMATION IN CONVERSATIONS:

Answers various questions during a conversation, including no/yes questions as well as wh questions and more complex questions. It is evaluated through watching.

Paraphrases information. The child is able to listen to new information and then recite the information back to them in their own language. This is measured by watching.

Correct responses to remarks. In conversation Do your child make remarks that don't make sense? It is a matter of watching.

Chapter 4: Grade Level-Listening Skills

As with all language abilities The complexity of language skills increases as your child grows older. In light of that I've put together this list of abilities related to grade levels. If you look through the list, you'll notice that a majority of the abilities are closely related to writing and reading. This is because writing and reading are all language-related skills, not just academic ones.

The hierarchy of the development of language skills is in the order of listening first and speaking next, followed by reading, and finally writing. The more skilled your child is in the lower levels the more successful they'll be in the higher levels.

Listening skills are essential for your child's academic progress. Each level builds upon the previous one. If your child is currently in the first grade, but has some difficulties with Kindergarten skills, start at the kindergarten level and work to master the first grade abilities.

Kindergarten

Reads stories, poems and even songs

Listening skills that are appropriate within groups

Answers on-topic questions when asked questions

Follows one step instructions

Answers yes/no questions

Answers to WH-type questions (who/what/where)

Completes easy Cloze responses (A dog can do ____)

Retells 3-4 incidents from a tale

It distinguishes between the same as well as different words (dog/doll)

Recognize rhyming patterns and words

The ability to rhyme can be used for example, like the frog and dog

Recognition of the word's number of syllables (clapping or snapping fingers)

Sound-symbol correspondence (knows letters and the sounds that correspond)

Sound Mix CVC words (d..o--g transforms into dog)

Can be segmented CVC words (dog becomes d..o..g)

FIRST GRADE

Appropriate eye contact

Needs clarification

Can repeat directions

Follow the 2 step instructions

Recalls details of the story (3-4)

Answer WH questions (who/what/where/when)

Sequence Four events

Finds the beginning and end vowels of words

The correspondence between sound symbols and

Blends (st; Blends (st; ...)

Long vowels

Short vowels

Can sound blend up to 2-4 phonemes into the word (w..a..t..er)

It can translate the simplest words in sounds (water turns into w..a..t..er)

You can add, remove or modify sounds to create new words (dog changes into doll)

SECOND GRADE

Follow 3 steps to get directions.

Needs clarification when they are not sure

Requests repetition

Can you recall specifics of the story?

Characters

Setting

Events

IDs primary idea following watching an audio presentation

Can you sequence events in a particular order? (3-5)

It identifies sounds at the middle, beginning, and ending of words

Can sound mix different phonemes in a word (b-a-n-a-n-a)

Can translate the simplest words to sounds (Banana transforms into b..a..n..a..n..a

THIRD GRADE

Follows complicated directions

Responds in a timely manner to comments from others and suggestions

Provides main idea and additional information

Determines the purpose of presentation

Answers WH questions (why/how)

Recapitulates story or details

Predicts future events based on a stories or data

GRADES 4-7

Responds to specific questions following listening to the experience

Responds to other's comments with a sense of propriety

Summary of the main concepts

Draws conclusions

Is it possible to discern between fact and opinion

Predicts based on the information provided

GRADES 8-12

Checks messages to ensure clarity

Sorting out and organizing important data

Draws logic inferences

Each school district and state has its own distinct goals and goals. If you'd like to be sure that you're focused on the things your school district believes is important, inquire about specific goals or goals. The state's website for education is an additional resource, as the goals and objectives are derived from the state.

Chapter 5: Strategies And Activities

We're now in the fun part! It's time to improve the listening skills of your child. The next question is what do you need to do to improve your child's listening abilities. One approach is to schedule a time with your child to are seated at an area and participate in various exercises. Also, it could be an hour of speech therapy. If you choose this option, I'd suggest that you attend at least two sessions per week, lasting 15 to 20 minutes.

Another option is to pick various games and activities to "play" together with the child. Do you have multiple children? You can let the children play. The more fun, the better. It doesn't matter what, any combination of both is also possible.

In this article, we'll talk about two different ways of developing or improving language capabilities, which includes listening skills. There's the top-down method and the bottom-up method.

The bottom-up method is the one where you examine an entire set of knowledge or learning goals and impart it to your child. For instance, if you would like your child to learn the alphabet, you can sit down and go through the alphabet repeatedly and over. Parents have been doing this for a long time with their children, and it has worked. Each of the activities listed in the checklists from the preceding chapters can be used to build specific skills by using the bottom-up method.

The top-down method is when you consider the language system as a whole. Making improvements to any part of your child's language or communication skills can have an impact on all individual abilities.

The top-down view is that the language abilities, including listening, are best acquired in the context of. The emphasis is on understanding the language in its entirety instead of specific skills.

As a speech pathologist that worked with students who were deaf or hard-of-hearing other speech pathologists often asked me what they could work on with a hearing-impaired child in their list of cases. I would say, "If you're talking with them, you're helping them develop their speaking abilities."

There's plenty of truth in this statement. Of course, I'd add more specific about these. Also when your child utilizes languages, the better they'll be in all aspects of speaking, which includes listening skills.

Both methods are effective. There is no advantage to one over the other. Actually, a mix of both is the most effective way to improve your child's listening abilities. Certain skills are best taught using a bottom-up method for example, the alphabet. Other skills can be taught using a top-down method including responding to a variety of questions.

Whatever age you are regardless of age, it is essential to start at the level that your child is at. This is why I suggest using checklists to provide you with an understanding of your child's strengths and weaknesses.

ATTITUDE RULES!

Whatever approach you choose to take the environment you create while learning the abilities is essential! It is important to create a positive atmosphere "speech therapy" session should be enjoyable for both you and your child.

Our attitudes and actions are a source of consequences. The creation of a safe and fun atmosphere for learning is much more crucial than the actual lessons themselves. In that regard, here are a few tips to be aware of that you should not forget, not just in the "speech therapy" time, but all the time.

Respect others. This is essential when you communicate with other people. Be respectful and hope that they also show respect to you.

Be open to other topics and topics. It is not a good idea to talk to people who only like to talk about themselves. Be attentive and listen to what people are looking to talk about, and they'll be more inclined to chat with you.

Be aware of your surroundings' non-verbal communications. Be attentive. If they're staring at their watches and are not looking at their watch, they may should leave, but aren't polite enough to disturb you. If they're looking at people around them they are probably bored them.

Be aware of the use of your private space. It is not pleasant to have people intruding into your privacy, so be mindful of this when communicating with other people.

Be nice. People love to talk to pleasant people. It's that easy, so try to be as friendly as you can. The old saying, "You can attract more insects with honey, is incredibly applicable when speaking with other people.

Be patient. If people think you're impatient and don't want to speak with them, they'll start to steer clear of them. Sooner or later you'll have no one who wants to speak with you.

Be optimistic. Of course, there will be moments and people who you might wish to vent with but you shouldn't be a victim of it constantly. Someone who just is a nice person to meet at the store does not want to hear of your headache or the fact that you're sick with your kid, or the fact that your dog wandered off!

Use appropriate eye contact. Do not use extremes with this issue. I don't want you cause a hole to the person with whom you're talking to by staring at them without blinking. However, I don't want you to never glance at them.

Take note of personal sound of your voice. This is a huge issue. For me, at least I can tell it's. Your voice can be sending messages that aren't trying to convey. If your voice is angry or sad, people will hear it regardless of what you convey.

Be aware of your own non-verbal communications. Be mindful of the messages your body transmits to your friend or partner in conversation. Your words could mean the same thing, however your body might be transmitting another thing.

Be open to understanding the viewpoint of your opponent. There are times when you may not be in agreement with someone, but If you are able to grasp the perspective of their viewpoint that will help keep the lines of communication open.

In the same way that our attitude and actions can encourage communication, the reverse is also true. Here are a few factors that could hinder communication. Here's a list with no-no's to remember.

Interrupting. There are times where you must interrupt, but when you perform it on a regular basis, you're sending an email to the person you are interrupting. You're telling them that you don't care what they're saying. You are telling them that it's only important that you be the one to speak.

Criticizing. If you're fast to criticize other people and then don't become the person people go to when they want to discuss a dilemma or a difficult situation. There are instances where people simply need to talk about their issues before they can resolve the issue.

Name calling. It's not ok to make a call to someone else's name. I don't care about what they did. I don't care about what your relationship with them is. It's not acceptable.

This will end to all their efforts to convey and comprehend your perspective.

Then you can tell them what they feel. People don't want to share how you are feeling or what you think about something. Sometimes, they would like to feel that you can understand the way they feel.

The idea of directing them to do something. This can work well when children are still young, but the older they get , the less effective it becomes. Communication is crucial. The act of directing the recipient to perform a task hinders the flow of communication.

Threatening. This can immediately stop the flow of communication. You might win that particular battle against the threats, but it does not close the doors to new opportunities to communicate in the future.

Making judgments about other people. We all have a tendency to judge others and their behavior and opinions. Human nature is a factor, but in order to keep your communication flowing, do not share your thoughts about judgment with people. Be quiet about it. However, this isn't necessarily the case for your children. It's your responsibility to evaluate their behavior and assist them in developing positive behaviors.

Too many questions. You're trying to ask questions, but If you ask many questions, you'll create a negative impression on your conversation partner. They might feel that you're being too private or curious. However, this isn't with your kids with regards to their activities outside. Get them involved! !

Talking about yourself only or your hobbies. People would like to hear about your story, but they'd prefer to speak about themselves. Let them have a conversation about themselves.

Blaming. Like accusing and judging the other person, blaming them isn't going to get you anywhere. It's possible that you are right, but it prevents anyone else from sharing their ideas or thoughts with you.

Utilizing a language that you are not familiar with. Avoid displaying pride when speaking with others. Use words they recognize.

Talking too fast. Do not make it difficult for those around you to speak to them. Talk in a manner that allows them to comprehend your thoughts.

Discriminating others by using code. I've experienced this and I'm sure many of you have too. In a situation in which everyone is discussing an issue that you have little about.

It's not a good idea to engage in this. An excellent example is when two people talk in a language that is different to the one used by others in the room, if they both speak the same language. It's unprofessional! Don't do it.

I'm sure there were some or two of the behaviors you either do or don't perform in the context of the previous actions. Do not worry about it. There is no way to be perfect. If you have observed something that you want to change, just select one of them and begin changing your own communications habits.

Children learn by the way they experience. Learning to communicate effectively can go a long way to ensure that your child is taught to communicate effectively that are both expressive and receptive (listening) abilities in language.

Strategies

Strategies aren't specific tasks however, they are things you can do regularly while you engage and interact with your children. Strategies can help strengthen their listening abilities and other communication abilities. Be aware that in any situation where the communication process is taking place and listening skills are being utilized. If you're speaking with your child, they are listening. Or they ought to be!

CHUNKING

It can be more easy for young children to understand information in chunks instead of individual words or the entire sentence. If you provide information, make sure to break it down into chunks that make sense.

For instance: The child was out to the market together with his brother.

Students are able to think about information in a manner which is understandable and, when you ask them questions they will be in a position to answer. What was the name of the boy who was running? What was the location where the child heading? Who was there with the boy?

This is particularly helpful when you are giving your child a set of instructions they must follow. The repetition of the words will help them keep track of the directions.

PARAPHRASING

Paraphrasing means saying the same information but in another way. If your child is confused over something you've said then try to explain it in another method. It is helpful to simplify it or explaining a certain word that you utilized that they don't have heard of.

For example you might say:

Take me to the cardinal's car and pick up my cell phone Please.

You're not the only one who can't help but look at you. It's time to. It's the right time to

Take me to the red car, and take my cellphone Please.

The first method was incorrect in fact I'd suggest to employ various words and grammar to help introduce your child to a more complex languages. However, if they look like they don't comprehend, try simplifying it to them.

CHECKING THEIR COMPREHENSION

If your child has trouble understanding language, make the habit of testing their comprehension. Have them repeat what you've said is one method to accomplish this. Another method is to ask them questions regarding the details.

The benefit of doing this is that the more you practice it the more your child will "tune to" to the words you're using because they know that you'll have them repeat the phrase.

ASK WHY ASK WHAT

Wh questions refer to who, what, when; where and the way. Questions on Wh are at higher than no/yes questions. For instance, when you're talking about your child's experience in school don't simply inquire, "did you have a great morning?" but rather ask, "What was the best aspect of your day? Or the most difficult?"

When you ask questions give them the possibility to discuss more, but they also won't be absorbed and respond by simply saying"yes or no.

Profiting from opportunities

While the two of you are going through your day There are a myriad of opportunities that appear that will allow you to develop your child's listening and language skills. Make use of these opportunities!

Here are a few examples:

While watching television While watching TV, ask your child describe what transpired in the program when the show was on commercial. This way, it's not just boring watching TV.

In the car take a few of the listening games that are listed in the section on activities.

When you read with your kid, do it to engage them in listening. You can ask them to answer questions on the book you're reading.

SONGS, NURSERY RHYMES AND FAIRY TALE

This category is one that I think merits a bit more focus. In the past, parents engaged in these kinds of activities simply because they were enjoyable! They did not realize they were enhancing the child's communication and listening skills , however, they were.

And not only that, there's a term that's called "cultural literacy." The concept of culture literacy is "things" that we can easily identify due to the culture that we are living in. A lot of these concepts and concepts are mentioned in the books we read. If your child is already familiar with the tale about Goldilocks along with The Three Bears, it will be much easier for the teacher when he speaks about Goldilocks in a different context for example, like the fact that it's illegal to take something from someone else. If they aren't sure who Goldilocks is and what it means, they'll get confused.

In addition to the development of cultural literacy, these programs are also designed to improve a range of language skills, such as intonation vocabulary, articulation and listening skills as well as expressive language.

They're also enjoyable!

MODELING

Did you remember when I said that your parents were the primary and most effective language teachers? It's true. Your child is listening and watching to you constantly. This is how they learn. If you're practicing good listening and speaking skills the child is developing good listening and communication skills.

Children learn from what they experience.

Let your child read to you!

The advantages from reading books to children regularly are numerous. Most importantly it will instill the love of reading and will help create a love of books that last for a lifetime. Additionally it will help improve your child's reading and listening abilities as well as expand their understanding of the world.

When should you begin with your kid's reading? Right now! It's never too early nor too late to begin with reading. What's more relaxing than reading a story to them while they lie upon your lap?

ACTIVITIES

This section might be renamed Games! Games! Games! Games are an excellent method to develop various language skills that include listening. They are entertaining and stimulating, and it's also an ideal way to build bonds with your child or children.

Some activities have particular goals, while others employ the more top-down approach. Keep in mind that both methods are effective. It's all about your child's strength and weakness, as well as the specific skills you're targeting.

BARRIER GAMES

Games for barriers can be played at any time and to develop a range of skill levels. I've played them with children in preschool as well as high schoolers. Barrier games are referred to as barriers because they create barriers between the listener and speaker, so they don't observe each other's behavior. A simple folder of files can sit between them in order that neither can see what they're doing to each other.

The idea is that the speaker provide directions while the listener tries to recreate a particular pattern. After the speaker has finished with the pattern, the barrier will be removed and the two people compare to see how well both did.

It could be a pencil and paper exercise. I would recommend that kids draw a line across and across, giving four blocks. Be sure that everyone who is playing gets a chance to talk to hear the speaker as well as the listener.

Beginning with simple, gradually becoming more complex as your child grows. Here are some suggestions:

Draw circles. Place two lines inside the circle.

Draw an outline of a circle. Place a line beneath the circle. Draw a square within the circle.

Draw 3 circles. Draw a line underneath one of the circles.

As you can see, you are able to help students learn vocabulary and concepts as you work on listening skills. Are you finding it too easy? You can add 3 or 4 different colors of crayons and it becomes more complicated.

It can also be combined with small toys or labels to create more entertaining for kids who are young. Your only limitation is your imagination in this exercise. Of course, the older your child gets the more complex the patterns are expected to be.

BINGO-TYPE GAMES

Everyone loves playing bingo games! And if you've got number of prizes to giveaway, that's even better. This game can be played to improve many different skills. It Is particularly good for improving listening abilities. Naturally, this means that the player talks, not showing the card. In the beginning you might have to do both, but gradually reduce the visual cues, and let your child depend on their ears.

I've added a blank bingo page at the end the chapter. (This could also be used for games that are barrier-free.) The only limit is your imagination as to the targets you can choose.

It's as simple or complicated as you'd like, depending on the age of your child. Here are a few examples:

The basic concepts of in the following categories: on; under and over. below.

Vocabulary: math, fairy tales, science Social studies and holidays

Simple math (you answer a question like 2 . you put a chip in the answer.

GAMES FOR COMMERCIAL

Don't worry I'm not talking about video games! I'm talking about games in which both the child and you are required to communicate and listen to each one another. Card games such as Go Fish or Old Maid are excellent when they allow you to speak and not only play with the cards. More intricate games like Candy Land, Monopoly are also great. Be sure to plan it in a way that they need to listen and talk, not simply play.

SOUND ASSOCIATION

Make sure your child is paying interest on specific sounds and then match them with the origin for the sounds. For example: cars/planes/trains/ambulances/fire trains/musical instruments.

Discriminates Sound Features

Utilizing musical instruments, help your children identify the following.

Loud/Soft

High/Low

Voiced/Voiceless

While playing the instruments, let your child watch and copy your patterns. Three long blows and one quick blow.

SPEAK SOUNDS ARE DISCRIMINATED

Hearing discrimination refers to the capacity to identify phonemes or sound. Your child should be able recognize the proper pronunciation of desired phonemes. After you have assessed this skill on the checklist, practice the sounds your child was having difficulty with.

Make up SMILEY, FROWN and SMILEY cards, or YES and NO cards. Children younger than 5 can use these cards to show the correct and incorrect sound. If they are older, the children might simply want to show whether they are right or wrong. The bells or buzzers could be used to increase the interest and excitement to the task.

1. Begin by explaining to your child the sound is.

2. Then you can play the sound again in isolation, by alternating it with other sounds that aren't like the target sound until the child can hear it for 90-100 percent all the time.

3. Repeat the process with the syllables, and later in words.

4. Start the process over again with similar sounds, in the same order that is isolated, words,, and words.

SOUND BLEEDING

Sound-blending Skills are the ability to recognize different sounds and create a word and then assign meaning to the word. This is a vital ability to be able to read. When your child is learning how to read, they need to be able to connect the words back together into the word.

In order to work to improve this ability, you can make use of a set of images to aid your child.

Place several images down and then repeat the sounds and help your child recognize the appropriate image.

Banana is now ba-na-na.

SEGMENTING AUDITORY

Auditory Segmenting Skills refers to the ability to comprehend the word and break it into smaller chunks of sound. This is an essential skill to be able to read. In the event that your kid is experiencing trouble reading, it might be beneficial to employ the visual aids that can help develop this skill.

Set up three blocks or chips in a row, each representing the word. Offer several examples and then take a touch or pick up the correct block each time you pronounce the sounds of the word. Choose words that have only 3 sounds initially but as your child gets better, make use of words that contain more than one sound.

Auditory segmentation is more challenging in comparison to sound blends for the majority of children. Therefore, you should work on sound blending first , and then work on auditory segmentation after your child is able to sound blend.

ALPHABET SOUNDS

Make sure your child is familiar with the sounds that go to each letter in the alphabet. Together, you and your child could cut pictures from magazines and create an Alphabet chart or book to work on learning the sounds.

There are a lot of fantastic ABC books available to study and master this ability. Children generally love learning their ABCs. Let them have fun learning it.

HOT SEAT

Place your child in the seat! Give them a flash card. They must name the letter and the sound and then provide an expression that begins with the letter.

A is aaa. The word "a" is used to describe Apple

They'll then place your name in the Hot Seat.

SOUND TRAIN

The purpose to the game to get your child to create the word that starts with the letter that is the final of the word that preceded it. The game is played using the Spelling Bee format It may be beneficial to write the last sound down so that they grasp the idea behind the game.

When you use the word "cat" Then they have to think of an adjective that begins at T. This aids in the awareness of sound's position as well as the sound-symbol correlation.

Skills in RHYMING

Kids love playing with words. When you both have some time shout out words and then ask them to create rhyming phrases. The Dr. Suess books are a fantastic way to practice Rhyming skills since we all are aware they are a great source of information. The Cat in the Hat is a master of That!

CLUE

Show the child images of everyday items, but in the end, they'll be capable of coming up with their own ideas. Ask them to describe about three or four different features of the object. Then, they will listen while you provide the clues.

It's a great way to relax in the car.

For instance: There's an animal that is in a zoo and has spots, and has a long neck. What exactly is it?

SCRAMBLED Sentences

Another way to get your hands dirty with words. It aids in listening and also with grammar.

CLOZE PROCEDURE -- FILL IN THE BLANKS

There's another option to get kids to play with words. Ask your child to complete the gaps by using the words and phrases they think are logical. Here are a few examples, but you are able to make any number of your own.

PHRASES:

_____ dog

_____ day

_____ hat

_____ tree

House _____

_____ girl

refers to what? _____

tall tall

red red

Sour _____

Sweet sweet _____

CLOZE SENTENCES:

I like eating _____.

I love to play _____.

There was a _____ in the Zoo.

The school is _____.

It's hot.

"___ is cold..

I'd prefer to _____.

_____ is simple.

_____ is big.

The car is _____.

My personal favorite game is _____.

Bears are _____.

ANTONYMS:

Make a statement and then ask your child to tell you the opposite of the word. This is also great to do in a car or while waiting for someone. It helps in processing language however it also helps to improve the ability to speak. Also, make as many of them as you require or desire.

UP/DOWN

HOT/COLD

SIT/STAND

BIG/LITTLE

HAPPY/SAD

GOOD/BAD

QUIET/NOISY

PRETTY/UGLY

LONG/SHORT

WET/DRY

SYNONYMS:

Same with antonyms.

WOMAN/LADY

MAN/GENTLEMAN

HAPPY/GLAD

SMILE/GRIN

CAR/AUTOMOBILE

ANGRY/MAD

CAT/KITTEN

FRIENDLY/NICE

MEAN/NASTY

IMPOLITE/RUDE

SIMILARITIES/DIFFERENCES

Tell your child what two things are the same, and also how they're different. This is a great way to develop thinking skills as well as for increasing the ability to communicate.

PIG/COW

FISH/SEAWEED

FINGER/TOES

NECKLACE/BRACELET

HAT/GLOVES

CAR/BIKE

SUN/BANANA

WATER/JUICE

CAKE/SUGAR

CAR/BIKE

ABSURDITIES

Write a funny line and ask your child to be able to explain the reason why it's so funny.

The cat is barking.

Lemons are delicious.

I am wearing a coat when it gets very hot.

Follow the directions below.

Begin with simple directions before you begin making them more difficult. When you've got some time to spare you can begin to give instructions. These could be in the form of actions or you could employ the format of a barrier game.

SIMON SAYS AND SIMON SILLY SAYS

The kids are in love with these. Are you looking to make it more challenging? Include music. So the child doesn't have several things to focus on but they must be focused on the words you say.

Silly Simon Says is similar to Simon Says. Students should adhere to the guidelines of the teacher . However, the teacher must say and do the same thing at times but at other times, perform something completely different from what is stated. Students are not in the classroom if they follow the instructions of the teacher does , not what she tells them.

TWENTY QUESTIONS

Imagine an object. The other participants take turns asking questions to provide more details. Questions must be yes/no questions. The winner will be able to choose the their next task.

TONGUE TWISTERS

They are enjoyable and children require your auditory memories to make sure they are correct. They also aid in language and grammar skills also. You can't beat this!

For instance:

Sally sells seashells on the beach.

Baby buggy bumpers made of rubber.

NURSERY RHYMES and SONGS

These programs help to improve listening and expressive language abilities. Additionally, it improves the literacy abilities of your child.

Jack Be Nimble

Humpty Dumpty

Mary Had a Little Lamb

TELLING STORIES

Story telling is a fantastic method of improving your language proficiency, and all languages. This is especially true to improve listening skills too. The art of storytelling can be accomplished through telling the tale. Or you could use illustrations or books for making it visually appealing to your kid. There are many different methods to use storytelling to help develop listening skills. These begin with simpler tasks and then become more challenging.

Answer the questions with a yes or no answer either during or following the story

Answer who/what/where/when/why questions during or after the story

First, what happened? then...

Find the characters.

Do you have a story to tell about something that each character did.

Retell the story

RIDDLES

Riddles are a fantastic method to increase comprehension. There are a lot of riddle books available. You can ask your librarian for guide you to one that's appropriate for your age. Here are some ideas to transform riddles into an game

Who am I? Provide clues to describe the person you are talking about. Example: I work in an educational institution, however I don't teach kids. I do however observe those who don't feel well. NURSE.

Where am I? Provide clues to describe locations. It's a place where you can see a doctor when you fracture your arm. HOSPITAL.

What do I mean? I'm an oak tree. My skin is yellow, but I'm also not round. BANANA.

What am I doing? The first step is to put something in an ice cube. I add water and eggs and mix it all together and place it into an oven. BAKE A CAKE.

YES/NO QUESTIONS. You can ask a range of questions which are both silly and serious.

Do you put on mittens in the summer?

Do dogs have more volume than cats?

Do you put on an outfit for bathing in the summer?

Do you wear clothes to eat?

Do you have the ability to take a dip in the ocean?

Are you outside?

Are you a boy(girl)?

Do you enjoy ice cream?

Can dogs bark?

Can a kangaroo run higher than cats?

Are you taller than your mother?

Do you have a higher age than mom?

Are bears more risky than the cat?

Is an airplane more loud than an automobile?

Are women more are taller than men?

Do lions and dogs have more power?

Are grapefruits larger than oranges?

WHY QUESTIONS. You can ask a variety of questions. Some are silly as well as some more serious.

What is the name of your instructor?

What time of day is it?

What are you most fond of eating? consume?

What are you doing at school?

What color is the sun?

Who's your best friend?

What is that chair?

What is your name?

Are you over the age of 65?

What will be your birthday?

What are you most interested in playing? do?

Where can you locate an ophthalmologist?

Why do you put on coats?

What time is Christmas?

Did you manage to make it there to school this morning?

When do you go your bed?

Where do you get to sleep?

Why do you want to go to your bed?

What time do you take your food?

What is the reason you consume food?

How do you get to school?

What is the reason you attend school?

What time do you start going to school?

What are you not allowed to take in?

What isn't there?

PAM Strategy. Present-Ask-Model.

This is a great way to do homework help in the absence of any specific task to tackle. Utilize a newspaper, book or magazine to gather an idea of a story.

1. Information currently available.

2. Ask questions about comprehension.

3. If the child isn't able to answer, read the information again by putting pressure on the information that can answer the question. If they are still unable to provide details, ask their parent for a gives a model answer.

4. Student repeats the answer.

The technique above is successful. It's not fast and may be frustrating but it also gives your child to hear the information, analyze the information, respond to questions regarding the information and then tell the story.

The key is repetition. this exercise.

CARDS FOR FOLLOWING DIRECTIONS. Similar to barrier games, but with index cards with a range of lines and shapes. Define the picture and then have students make copies of the image. Make sure you include prepositional phrases into your descriptions.

Complexity is determined by the level of language and age of students. Once they are proficient at a the appropriate level, they can be allowed to explain pictures to you or to someone else to help with the development of expressive language.

Examples of prepositions include: in, on, under between; top middle; bottom; first, second; beginning and ending.

Finding the main IDEA. Listen to the material in a way that is appropriate for their age. Then , ask them to tell the basic concept. The use of text books or reading books is the ideal way to teach this ability.

Imagine a story. Tell a story (3-4 principal events) and then ask your child to follow play the stories in order. This is an excellent method to use at any age.

Fairy tales and nursery rhymes are fun ways to engage in this kind of activity. Rehearse the nursery rhyme a few times and then ask your child draw the rhyme. Cut a piece of paper into four pieces and let them get imaginative. Once they've finished drawing it then ask them to retell the story.

Jack and Jill were on their way to the top of the mountain. Jack fell and injured his crown. Jill was thrown to the ground.

Here's an example for the older children:

The Pilgrims arrived in America in 1620 aboard a vessel called the Mayflower to enjoy freedom of religion. They made their way to Plymouth Rock which later became part of Massachusetts. It was a winter that proved challenging and many people got sick, and some even passed away. In the spring of the year, the Indians began to make close to the Pilgrims and taught how to plant corn, as well as other crops. In the fall, they created a special day to express gratitude to God for their new friends and their home. The day was dubbed Thanksgiving.

As you can observe, there are plenty of methods to focus on developing your child's ability to listen. There's no reason for them to be bored.

Something I didn't talk about but I'd like to mention is homework. Consider homework for your child as an opportunity to improve the listening abilities of your child. This will aid students in school too.

For instance, take the story they're working on this week. Let them read it Ask them questions about the story along with the character. Talk about words that are unfamiliar to the children. Read it out loud to them over and over again.

This will allow them to be successful in school and increase their listening skills in the process. This method can be applied for any subject. You can read the science book with them and ask questions , or social studies or anything else.

Additionally, as you go about this, you'll begin to know your child's strengths and weaknesses the area of interest. This can give you more suggestions on how you can assist your child at school.

Don't not forget that you read with your kid to have amusement!

Chapter 6: Speech And Language Development
Our first chapter was focused at child development generally We are currently focusing more specifically on language and speech development, and some of the problems that could be encountered. A lot of children don't speak until they reach the age of five years old. However, it's the time from birth to age three that's most critical in a child's speech as well as language development. This is the time that is a time of rapid maturation of the brain and , in particular the capacity to learn the ability to speak and communicate. We've heard of the brains of toddlers being likened to sponges, which is definitely the case. The more exposure you give your child to language in this stage and the more easy it will be for them to. There are children who suffer from language or speech issues who will not attain these milestones, no matter how much language they're exposed to.

Disorders of speech and language tend to be considered to be one in the same, however there's a distinction. When we speak of an issue with language, we mean problems children experience in comprehending what people are saying or communicating their feelings. However children who are struggling with syllables, sounds and words, or even a stutter may be diagnosed with an issue with speech sounds.

There's been plenty of controversy over the words 'developmental language disorder' (DLD) and 'specific language impairment' (SLI). Many people, both professional and non-professional, are using them interchangeably, and a lot of research you've read does not define a distinct distinction. We'll remain with the term DLD since many people will believe that SLI is extremely specific and it is more likely children's difficulties with language and speech are due to other ailments and not just one. In the UK the term'speech, communication, and language requirements' (SLCN) is widely used.

Bilingual Speech

With the increasing number of immigrants and movement, it's more typical for children to grow to live in multilingual environments. This raises the question of whether children who have difficulties with speech or language should be exposed to a different language.

How do you allow your kid to learn more than one? Should you even try to do so, if you've discovered an LD? Then things are likely to become a bit more difficult however, nothing is impossible! It is important to keep in the mind that speech and language research is still fairly new and the same could be said about the concept of bilingualism. We are aware that children who are bilingual achieve higher academic results and improved language use in social settings and greater cognitive ability to adapt. There's not enough research to show the long-term benefits of children who are learning two or more languages , while dealing with delays in speech and language or other issues.

Let's take a look at two sides to the debate. Many believe it is the case that, if your child is having issues with one language, it will be more difficult to master the second. Because of this, parents are advised to use their native language at home. Or in the case that they speak multiple languages at home and want to stick one parent one language' principle that each parent uses only one language to their child. However you can benefit from the early years, in which the brain is absorbent, allows children to a wider range of vocabulary. At this point they're also not worried about the fact there are two language options to learn. This isn't like us adults who need to translate and investigate every grammatical pattern! Children listen and learn. However returning to the beginning idea, children who have problems with language and speech will not be capable of listening and learning like others bilingual children do. In the end, the Multilingual: Empowering Individuals, Transforming Society project (MEITS) declares that reducing the amount of languages that a child suffering from difficulties with speech and language will not treat the condition. Instead of a child who is bilingual who suffers from speech and language issues, you're one who is monolingual and suffers from difficulties with language and speech. In addition, a bi- (or multilingual) child will be more likely to have difficulties with speech in all their languages in if they share the same sounds in speech. This can be the determining factor in determining what next steps to take.

One of the common reasons against encouraging bilingualism combination with speech and language issues is the availability of resources. It is logical that UK therapists have been trained to provide therapy in English and, as such you can expect treatment in English. However you should utilize your native language to work on your child's goals at home, particularly when your child isn't currently in school. When your child attends school, the same strategies are provided to the school staff to discuss together to ensure that the same level of support at home as well as in the school.

As a mother with experiences in both bilingualism and the development of speech and language I am able to give you the following tips. Take a look at all the advantages and disadvantages of your child's specific situation. Discuss the situation with your specialists in your group and seek as much knowledge from them as you can using the available resources. For instance, if you are using one of these play-based therapy methods and it is the one the experts recommend for your toddler it is logical to try the techniques in your native tongue in case that's the language you are most likely to use at home. If, however, your five-year-old is in school and have been assigned speech therapy to help develop their English language it is recommended to take the time to learn the techniques of therapy in English as well as try the techniques at your home. It is natural that the sessions take place in English however you should still utilize your native language at home for interactions and play to keep building the language at home. Every situation will be the same , and there isn't a definitive either or not answer to this question.

Receptive Language

Receptive language is the one we learn and comprehend. It is evident that the development of the language occurs at various levels.

12-18 months: Children is able to comprehend simple, information-carrying words or words. For example, if , for instance, you request your child of 15 months to take you to the remote for your TV then they'll be capable of comprehending. You might initially have to employ gestures to help your understanding. For instance, you could point at the remote and say "Get the remote. At this age can comprehend words you are likely to use regularly at home, such as eating, sleeping,or drink'. Children will be able to show the parts of their body when you call them. For example, "eyes" mouth, 'nose'.

3-4 years: Children begin to comprehend instructions that contain two words carrying information. For instance, 'Give the teddy a spoon it is in the case of an alternative between a dolly and teddy and a choice between the spoon and cup. Children will start to comprehend the purpose that everyday items serve. For instance, they'll be aware that scissors are to cut hair, a hairbrush to clean your hair, and a toothbrush for brushing your teeth.

Three to four years old: Kids be able to comprehend three words that convey information. For instance, 'Give Teddy an apple and one banana. For instructions to count as an explicit word, you need to provide a second alternative for your child to pick from or else all they need to do is take the item that is in the front of them. At this point children should be able to comprehend the concept of size such as 'big' and'. The children must also be able to recognize and identify various colours.

4 to 5 years At this stage children are able to comprehend instructions that contain four words carrying information. For instance, "Put the spoon in the drawer and the cup under the sink. This happens while the kid is at the kitchen and they can see the cup and the spoon as well as a few other items around them. Make sure you have other options in case it doesn't be considered a key word.

Expression Language

If a child is around two an age, they will be able to speak between 150 and 300 single-word phrases. I know what you're thinking, that's a lot of words! I guarantee you that should you just sit down one day and begin making notes, you'll be amazed by how quickly your normally growing child is absorbing the language.

But, I understand the reason why you purchased this book because your child isn't talking much in any way. We'll talk about that more in the next chapter.

If your child has the largest single-word vocabulary Start adding words to the single word. It is important to add a second word to the single word, and then say two words to the child. Your child should be able to engage in an informal conversation with you by using two-word phrases like"More juice 'Daddy car' or 'Go out My turn, etc.

The more you practice the language through repetition (correcting while not noticing you're correcting) more quickly they'll be able to master. For instance If your child is saying"Chair," you could say"Yes that's the chair of Daddy. When your kid is looking at you as you drive and says, "Mummy car', you can say, 'Yes, Mummy is in the driver's seat.'

We will go over the methods to increase understanding and communication in the section on therapies.

We've examined the development of language in the typical child. Let's take a take a look at some of the issues you might face. Your child could be delayed in language development - by the time they are two years old, they might only be able to speak 30 single words , and might not yet put words together to form two-word sentences. If there's no additional health concerns or health issues and your child is healthy, it is possible that they is continuing to develop their language skills , but they will require additional assistance from you.

Communication before Words

Get without your kids for a moment and contemplate our conversations without words. Imagine a time your friend ate a mouthful and then wildly waved at napkins or the store attendant who gave you the most warm smile. What is the expression of the person you love most, as you feel their affection towards you in their eye? It's not all about words. As parents (and I've been there) we are so focused on the stages of development and waiting for that important first word that our perception is clouded and perhaps our ears are stuck.

Communication begins much earlier than words. If a baby is crying it is a sign that something is not right. If you approach the baby and hear your voice, they become calmed. It could be a simple "There is my sweetheart, there's my love or "Dear me, I still need to take the dog for a walk and clean the bathroom.

Your voice, not your words that produce the calming effect.

What are the different stages of communication Before Words?

* Pre-intentional: This is when your child is smiling, vocalizing or mumbles, but there is no intention behind the message.

• Anticipatory Communication: The child is able to anticipate your response. Consider a game like a peek-aboo. You cover your face using your hands, then play with your hands, and then call out "Peek-aboo". If you repeat this practice often the baby will start to anticipate what you are doing and will look forward to it. They could be able to show this by smiling or waving their hands or arms before saying the words.

* Intentional communication Your child's hands or body in a way, makes a sound or performs an action such as tugging on your clothes, or using their hands to lead you to a place - they purposely would like something to happen or convey their thoughts or feelings.

* Ideas and words Words and ideas: Children learn to use words and will eventually make use of them to express their thoughts, opinions questions, and thoughts.

* Joining words and concepts the more vocabulary they learn the more likely they are to begin to join them in sentences to communicate themselves.

We've discussed the way that babies use pre-intentional and anticipatory communication. But, it is important to be aware that some children that are older may be experiencing pre-intentional stage because of their speech or disorder of speech, resulting from complicated medical conditions. It is important to focus your efforts towards helping them develop their abilities at their current stage of speech and language. Don't focus on their age , but rather at the level of understanding they have. If, for instance, your child is five years old, they are young, they may have more complex needs and their communication is anticipatory. Therefore, you should work to get them to the next stage, that is intentional communication rather than relying on words or thoughts as that's an immense leap. However, despite your excitement it is important to change your expectations.

The level of your communication skills will play a part. I have a friend who speaks so fast that I am unable to comprehend her. Another member of my family adds "like" in between each word. My grandmother was very articulate. I have heard of people who talk incredibly slow to children and babies or in such a loud volume that I'm convinced they've taken the air from an balloon made of helium. It is not necessary to get caught up in the frenzied process of teaching family members about the proper manner of speaking to your child. But, you should calmly remind them of the fact that there's no need to be a snob and that they need to use appropriate words to describe objects and utilize as many different words as is possible.

Communication involves listening and speaking - or in this case watching. See how babies react to various rhythms, sounds and rhythms. See the objects they point at and then listen to the first sounds of babbling that are created. When you speak, let them take the opportunity to talk in order to communicate in real life - talking and listening. As they grow older, they can use words to describe the objects they point at. There is no need for many expensive toys to help them develop the early stages of communication. Colors, textures, and sounds are essential. Saucepans wooden and plastic spoons dishescloths and sponges and odd socks stuffed with various materials are some ways to stimulate a baby's curiosity and help them develop vocabulary and communication prior to words.

There's many things that you could do in order to create an environment that is awash in communication prior to the first time your baby's words are spoken. One of the words that parents like is "routine" and with excellent reasons. Establishing a routine gives the chance to do repetitive routines. Repetition of activities can lead to repetition of vocabulary! We'll talk more about this as we explore the treatments you can perform at home.

Chapter 7: The Language Delays And Disorders

If you're taking a look at this text, it may be because you've got some concerns about the issues that your child may be experiencing with their communication. You could also find that you've received a diagnosis and want to seek further guidance. There's still a grey space between. Since every child is unique and needs to be able to find the most effective strategies for helping your child, it is necessary to get an assessment. I would advise against taking this book to read and taking matters in their own hands. Yes, I'm repeating myself, but that's what it is!

It can be a difficult moment for parents to find their child struggling in any way. The first thing people go towards is Internet however, there are so many abbreviations terminology and medical terms it can make them feel even more confused than they did when they first started. There is ample time learn the lingo related to the many different treatments and treatments, so let's take some time to review some of the phrases you'll encounter to make sure you're more comfortable with them, and also, be less scared by them.

What is the difference between a Disorder and a Delay?

The first thing to consider to ask is whether the child is suffering from an issue or is suffering from. As you could imagine that when we speak of the possibility of a delay in speech or language this means the child may be progressing in their development of language, but slowing down the pace than the other kids. They're achieving the crucial milestones, but not at the typical age. However a language or speech problem is the case when a child isn't acquiring the necessary skills or is learning them in an way that is considered to be abnormal.

What is the difference between Expressive and Receptive Language Disorders?

I like to think of it as "what's going into and out', but as therapy, I'll explain it in a more professional manner. It is crucial to note in this article that children develop the ability to comprehend the meaning of a language before they speak it. Receptive language disorders happen when children are unable to comprehend the meaning behind what is being spoken to them. They may be able to comprehend basics of instructions but they struggle to comprehend more complicated language, or not be able to comprehend even basics of Instructions. This could be in the sense of they don't understand the language, or they have issues regarding their hearing.

Expressive language delay occurs when your child is unable in communicating with you through either non-verbal or spoken language. Language disorders occur when children's language skills are developing , but not in a regular pattern. They may face difficulties when they're not able to express their emotions or desires. Remember that at 2 years of age, children enter an initial phase of frustration because they are aware of what they want , but do not have the abilities to communicate. The process is normal part of development, but can turn into an issue if it doesn't go away.

It's possible that children also have issues with both their receptive as well as expressive language. If you've ever been on vacation to an unfamiliar country and attempted ordering food in a different language you might be able to comprehend some of the frustration they experience.

The delays in speech and language and disorders can be linked to health issues. In the majority of cases children, they are healthy and bright. with the assistance of a qualified Speech and Language Therapist the right plan can be developed.

Developmental Language Disorder DLD

DLD is more prevalent than people think and is estimated to affect one in 15 children being diagnosed with it. It's a common name for children who struggle with comprehending and communicating. It could be due to difficulty in making the correct words, using appropriate grammaral structures or having a small vocabulary. Younger children might have difficulty remembering new words. As they grow older, it becomes difficult for them to comprehend that words may have multiple meanings, such as trees' bark or the bark of the bark of a dog. Children suffering from DLD may have difficulty describing what they feel in stories, or comprehend longer sentences. Though they are extremely intelligent, their struggles with language could cause issues with socializing and learning at school.

However, the precise reason behind DLD isn't known yet. It could be a result of genetics or cognitive, or environmental, or any combination of. The diagnosis is usually not made until after the age of school in which parents and teachers can begin to identify the issues that a child is experiencing. Because language is essential for every subject, you could see a lot of poor marks and less progress than kids who are in the same grade.

Making people aware of DLD can aid in early intervention and decrease the chance of children being without being diagnosed. There are many ways to find RADLD across the UK as a group consisting of educators, parents scientists, health professionals and researchers to educate the public about DLD.

Certain general red flags could include the inability to understand the language, a lack of gestures and the family history of impairment in language. In the case of the specific age group, DLD can appear in the following manner:

Age 1-2 years old

* Your child isn't using babble.

* They don't reply (with phrases) when you talk to them.

* They're not trying to contact you.

Age: 3 to 4 years old

* Your child has no language or signs.

They're not talking to you (with the words) when you try to talk to them.

* They could have used words before, but have stopped making use of them anymore or have stopped developing additional languages.

Age 3-4:

At this time your child is using two words.

* They're still having trouble understanding simple instructions.

The speech of your child isn't clear enough that even your family members have trouble understanding them.

* Other things you might notice are that your child is using jargon in place of words, echolalia or adult language instead of speaking in a spontaneous manner or being slow in developing verbs.

4 to 5 years old:

Their interactions could be inconsistent or irregular and they may not be able to comprehend.

* At this stage your child may be using three-word words.

The speech of your child will appear more distinct, and the entire family will be able comprehend about 50% of the time However, strangers will not be able to comprehend the speech of your child.

Age 5:

* Your child might have difficulty retelling an account or explain what they have learned at the school.

* They may struggle to comprehend what they've just read or heard.

* Your child might struggle to remember the instructions they were given to accomplish (recalling the instructions).

* Your child is able to talk often, but they're not great in to-and-fro conversations.

* They might interpret the information they hear literally , and they might not grasp the meaning of the information provided.

* Other things you might be able to notice is that they will employ sentences, but the words are not in the correct order.

A great methods that can be used is by making everything visually. Encourage your child to utilize visual aids to communicate their message through photos or drawings. Additionally, you should employ simple and consistent language that makes the process easier to comprehend.

What is the problem with Dyslexia?

While dyslexia is a disorder that affects written language it's still something speech and language therapy therapists are able to help with. People with dyslexia may have difficulty recognizing letters, words and other symbols. Reading may be difficult and it could be difficult in naming certain words. They might struggle with spelling and write certain numbers or letters in reverse. The speech and language therapy therapist may assist dyslexic children to increase their phonological awareness, specifically, things such as the rhyming process, segmenting and mixing words, and recognizing the beginning and ending sounds in words and manipulating the sound.

In addition to speech and language therapy should your child be experiencing signs of dyslexia, you may want to talk to the school about it and ask them to refer you towards an educator psychologist to conduct an evaluation. The psychologist who is studying education might suggest using colored overlays for reading time. These are films with transparent surfaces which can be layered over text to lessen the visual stress. It is essential to talk with your child's teacher in the event that they aren't aware of the difficulties your child is having in writing and reading. The guidance and support offered by the psychologist for education will have more impact on the child as well as the progress they will achieve. It is also important to mention that schools are governed by budgets and usually send children who have the most difficult issues. So, be ready for schools to refuse a referral even if your child's problems are not severe.

Chapter 8: Speech Sound Delays And Disorders

After we've clarified the distinction between disorder and delay and disorder, I will make use of the term "disorder" in general to facilitate reading. Every one of the problems with speech and language that I go into detail about are now viewed as a delay or disorder apart from those that are related to hearing. This list is not in any way in any way ordered by the severity. The sooner you get help, the best option If you're concerned or something rings an alarm bell, don't be hesitant to call your healthcare professional.

Articulation Disorders

Disorders of speech are when the child's speech sounds are developing , but not in the normal pattern. Children may mispronounce words for a longer time than they ought to. A good example is not putting sounds at the start and/or at the conclusion of phrases. For instance the child could say "do" instead of "dog and "bi" instead of "bike'. In contrast adding words is when children add an additional sound to the word. Instead of saying 'car', they could use "cart" or "buhlack", instead of black. The additions aren't as widespread as other problems with articulation. Some children make substitutions: they swap one sound for an untrue sound. "Very" can be pronounced as 'bery', and "red" as 'wed'.

If a child requires help by a sound distortion the reason is that they've got the majority of words right, however there could have some distortion. The most frequently sound distortions include /l/, /r and /s/. The sound /s/ could be made by the side of the mouth, rather than in the middle on the tongue. There is whistling sound "sheep" is spoken more like'shleep'.

Phonological Disorders

Disorders of speech are motor-based and the phonological disorders are neurologically-based. Family members may be able comprehend the child's speech, however others might not. Cluster reduction refers to groups of clustered sounds like /sn/ that are mispronounced, with the /s/ dropping completely. "Snap", "snail," and'snake' could be described in the form 'nap' and "nake". Another problem is the final consonant deletion. It is normal for children not to miss certain consonants, but they do they should all be deleted.

Velar forwarding as well as stopping are linked to sound and circulation of air. When you say "cat" and "gold" you'll notice that your tongue presses against the roof of your mouth toward the back, which hinders airflow. This happens in the case of /k/ andsound. Velar fronting implies that children cannot put their tongues in that the sounds are not pronounced. /k/ and /gsound are made in the form of /d/ or/, meaning that "cat" would be spoken as "tat". When we make fricative sounds, we require air flow to make the long sounds, in particular the sound /shor. "Sheep" is an extended initial sound. without air, children can substitute the /sh/ sound with the sound of a shorter one, such as using the words 'tip' or "pip'.

Apraxia

Within our brains, there have a set of muscles. These muscles allow connection between our speech functions and the brain. The term "apaxia" refers to the time the condition where these connections are broken or damaged. In spite of being aware of what they wish to say, the person cannot communicate this through words. This is why they are able to write what they'd like to write but, without the connection with the brain or speech organ, they're unable to communicate it verbally. The condition of Apraxia is caused by brain damage , but for children, the root cause isn't known.

Apraxia may be light or cause total incoherence. Since the lips, muscles or tongues aren't moving in the proper manner, children might not be able speak often or have difficulty in forming sounds and words. In the case of mild instances, it's difficult to distinguish Apraxia from other speech disorders. Apraxia symptoms for children include the inability to say words the same way every time, or making changes in the sounds. They often emphasize the wrong syllables in the word. Also, you may observe that words with shorter lengths are easier to pronounce . However, longer words can be difficult to pronounce.

Dyspraxia

Dyspraxia is a disorder that can affect planning and motor movements. It isn't only restricted to speech. To help clarify the difference between the two, we refer to it as "verbal dyspraxia" or "dyspraxia of speech' as dyspraxia can affect the limbs or the body. The most common signs of dyspraxia include a food-related issues or messy eating as well as a reduced concentration level, difficulty in keeping still, or to sit still. They may also be clumsy.

Verbal dyspraxia may manifest as a lack of speech during the first few months of life They will be able to speak with a sluggish speech by age three, and their development with speech will typically be slow. As with apraxia it is an illness caused by weakening in the muscles of speech. It may range from moderate to severe. Dyspraxia may be acquired (through an injury or illness) or it can be a result of developmental issues, manifesting in children.

A child who has dyspraxia of the voice may have difficulty to make words in the correct sequence to form words - especially with long complex, long words. It is possible that they be able to say a difficult word but be unable to repeat it correctly. Children often be slow to locate the word they would like to use. Another indication of dyspraxia with verbs is a monotone voice because it's difficult to use correctly stress and rhythms.

Auditory Processing Disorder (APD)

This disorder alters the communications between brains and ears. When sounds reach the ear, there's some sort of interference the time they reach the brain, which means that the sound won't be heard in the normal way. Children suffering from APD are unable to follow the conversation and distinguish sounds that occur between words. The issue is more severe when they're in noisy environments such as the classroom. It's not the same as an autistic child that is extremely sensitive to loud sounds.

APD symptoms aren't always apparent in the event that other speech and language problems are present. It is up to an audiologist as well as Speech and Language Therapists who will assist a child aid them in their the use of sound and speech therapy.

Hearing Loss

It's no surprise that a child suffering from hearing loss is likely be prone to major delays in development of speech and language The earlier hearing loss begins harder it gets. Hearing is essential for developing verbal language. We all know that children learn by watching and mimicking adults around them. If your child can't understand what you're speaking, they won't be able to replicate your words. It is essential to have your child's hearing examined whenever you observe that they aren't paying attention when you say their name, or when they are watching your mouth attentively while you speak, and, of course, in the event that your child is more than 12 months of age and isn't talking. Children can suffer from Ear infections that can be detrimental to hearing and they are more likely to experience delays in speech development.

After they've been examined and given the necessary treatment that should hopefully correct any issues they may have, they should be able to improve their speech and develop with a normal rhythm. But, they might require assistance from an audiologist or speech therapy.

In the UK hearing loss in children is checked before the time of birth. If you are concerned you should speak to your health professional or doctor. They will be capable of referring your child to an audiology department. They will determine the best treatment for your child and recommend appropriate options like grommets or hearing aids, based on the degree of the hearing loss of your child.

Speech sound issues are common in young children. Certain children learn the proper pronunciations by listening to adults around them or by doing one-on-one with their parents, which involves modeling and auditory stimulation, however we'll discuss this in the chapter on therapies.

Some children will require help from a professional, since the mistakes they're making must be corrected after a certain time. For instance, if your child who is six years old is making use of /t/ instead or /k/, or your child is still using "wion" instead of "lion or ', it's the right time to seek help from speech therapy. It's normal for a toddler to use 'wabbit' or "labbit" for "rabbit" however, it is not the case for a 7-year-old.

Children with hearing impairments are prone to hearing issues and making the 'quiet sound' like /s/ and /for. They also decrease specific cluster sounds like "spoon" is pronounced as 'poon', and'square may be made by "quare". A few mistakes are fairly common and every child makes them at some point as their speech sound system develops.

Certain children do not make the sounds at either the word's beginning (initial vowel sound) or at the end the word. As an example, you may see your child saying "be" to mean "bed" or 'oft' to mean soft. It is also possible to hear children remove a whole syllable from the beginning of the word - for instance, the word "banana" is often pronounced as "nana". This is also normal for children of a young age, however if your child is six and is generating words that sound like this, then it is time to seek out assistance from a professional.

Assistive Listening Devices

Audiologist can determine whether your child is in need of an assistive hearing device. There are three kinds of assistive devices that aid those with hearing loss or speech, voice as well as language issues. ASL devices (ALDs) can amplify sounds, especially when there is a lot of background noise. AAC and augmentative communication (AAC) devices assist users to communicate with others. AACs could be picture boards or may be more advanced like applications that convert text into speech. In addition, they connect to devices such as the doorbell or telephone and the light will flash to warn users.

Glue ear is a frequent disease that is seen in children, specifically those who have Down syndrome. The ear afflicted by glue is the result of a build- of fluids within the middle ear, and as a frequent issue, may affect language and speech. Grommets are plastic tubes that are placed into the eardrum to allow air to enter your middle ear. A doctor might suggest this procedure to treat persistent glue the ear or for an ear infection. Grommets are a temporary treatment and are expected to fall out on their own between six and 18 months following having been put in. This is enough time to allow the tubes between the middle ear and the eardrum to grow and function independently.

Chapter 9: The Conditions That Are Influenced

By Social Conditions

This may not always be the situation, but there could be some conditions that will be more pronounced in social settings. This can be quite a challenge for parents, since at home the language and speech don't appear to be as difficult. Your baby may be content talking to their parents and children, but once Auntie and uncle arrive the scene changes. Two things I caution against. The first is putting your child to engage in social activities in order to help them over come their handicap. The words, such as "It's only Auntie' or "Go ahead, go out and play with other kids' aren't likely to be helpful as it's not something they are able to manage. That brings me to my next point. Be wary of assuming the child shy. This is why I've detailed the milestones, what to expect, and when to talk to professionals.

Muteness/Selective Mutism

A child who is mute doesn't talk in any way. Selective mutism happens the condition where a child isn't able to talk in different situations. Parents need to be cautious when it comes to selective mutism as they often get frustrated when their child speaks in certain situations, but not in others. Sometimes, it can feel like they're being difficult or that they aren't doing enough. It's not about choosing not to speak, but about being unable to do so, which is mental disorder that stems from shyness and extreme anxiety. The diagnosis is made by the expertise of a group of experts comprising speech and language therapists as well as an education psychologist. A treatment plan can be developed together, as the child could also be suffering from the disorder of speech and language responsible for selective mutism.

ASD - Autism Spectrum Disorder

The autism spectrum is so wide and diversified, communication difficulties may range from being insignificant or not noticeable, to total withdrawal or the mutism. ASD children may struggle with language and speech development as well as tone of voice and non-verbal communication. The majority of the time the speech and language issues associated with ASD children cause problems in social interactions.

Language can be very repetitive and some ASD children suffering from a condition known as echolalia. They repeat the exact phrase or word immediately following hearing it, or delayed echolalia when they'll repeat it afterward. The vocabulary can be restricted in certain subjects, unless they are particularly interested in and, then, they'll possess a wide range of words.

Therapy for speech and language will assist a majority of ASD children develop the ability to communicate. There are however some children who do not have the speaking and language abilities. In these instances therapy will help the child to develop different ways of communicating, like gestures, symbol systems, or the use of sign language. You will find more details about ASD from my book 'Understanding Autism. Take a Mile in their Shoes'.

Is ASD and DLD related?

Both conditions overlap, however they also have distinct distinctions. It is rare to see repetitive behaviors when you have DLD. Unlike ASD the condition doesn't typically manifest with other conditions. ASD requires an official medical diagnosis. DLD is more likely to be recognized through a doctor, and more likely to be diagnosed by an educator. However both are lifelong illnesses that cause challenges in social situations, including expression of thoughts and feelings and comprehending speech and language.

Stutteringor stammering

Stuttering is a very common speech disorder, often referred to as stammering. You're probably aware that you might have experienced a stuttering moment usually when you're anxious, or when a particular situation could cause a stammer. In these instances it's not an issue in your everyday life, and it's not considered to be a sign of a speech disorder. Therapists for speech and language view it a disorder if it has a negative impact on daily life or when a person is unable to perform certain activities to prevent the possibility of stuttering. Stuttering could also be caused by due to a developmental issue or triggered by illness or injury, as well as psychological and emotional trauma.

The root of the stammering problem is unclear. It may be genetic because approximately two-thirds of people who stammer have a background of stammering. It may also be due to complexity of the process of developing speech. It's an extremely complicated process for the young brains and often the neural pathways are miswired or are not yet connected. About 66% of children will get rid of stammering. Alongside working on the emotions that trigger the stammer (fear or anxiety) an experienced Speech and Language

Therapist will develop an action plan to enhance your child's communication.

One thing that's going greatly help here and for which there is no need for therapy in the area of speech and language is confidence and love. Give your child a high-five and give them hugs and sweet words. Give them time to talk, but refrain from completing the sentences. Accept their struggles in speaking. Make sure that all members of the family have the chance to speak during family gatherings, including those with a stammer. The more you can help to accept their style of speaking, the more comfortable they'll become. However, some older children might require help by a specialist speech therapistwho can help both you and your school be aware of the issue and offer strategies for helping your child.

Chapter 10: Down Syndrome

The Down syndrome doesn't cause speech or language disorder since it's an illness on its own. However I'd like to talk about it because children suffering from Down syndrome are prone to developing problems with speech and language and also difficulties with social communication. This is a complicated topic due to the fact that Down syndrome is a spectrum that can differ in its severity and manifestations. It is imperative to adhere to the advice and guidance given by your specialist. It doesn't mean you should not use the techniques that are in this book, however for the best outcomes, your team can develop a well-organized program based on the specific requirements for your child.

Down syndrome was named for the English doctor John Langdon Down. While Down syndrome was known for many centuries however It was Down who came up with the first exact description. The people who suffer from Down syndrome are born with an additional chromosome. Instead of 46 chromosomes inside each cell they have 47 with the 21st one being duplicated. Down syndrome can result in physical and mental disability, however due to advancements in research and the understanding of society of the condition, a lot of adults are able to live a full and satisfying life. This is especially helped through early interventions.

Concerns with speech and language are more likely to result in problems rather than delays in children who suffer from Down syndrome. But that doesn't claim that every child won't suffer from issues also. A second general rule is that children who have Down syndrome are more receptive to abilities in language than expressive ones. This is due to the fact that they can understand but struggle with grammar and the tenses.

Another aspect to take into consideration with Down syndrome and the development of speech and language is the effect of hearing problems which many children have. Children who have Down syndrome have smaller and more narrow ear canals when compared to other children. This could result in more infections in the ear, which can result in a decrease or total loss of hearing. Hearing loss is a frequent issue that can impact a child's ability to understand the spoken word and speak as a crucial element of development.

It is possible to find a connection between children suffering from Down syndrome as well as working memory. The disorder means there is a problem with the loop of phonology. This loop allows us to recall the sound patterns and connect words to their significance. The impairment isn't affecting the visual short-term memory. That is the reason visual aids are extremely helpful.

Children who have Down syndrome may have difficulty in making speech sounds since the disorder alters the facial structures, nerves, and muscles. Three factors that hinder oral motor function are smaller mouth cavities, bigger tongues, and a more arched palate. You've heard me before and you'll know that I'm not saying that this is identical for all children who suffer from Down syndrome. Like not all boys who suffer from Down syndrome experience difficulties with the structure of their mouths and larynx. These are but a few of the physical reasons for speech and language problems and delays.

It is also estimated to be 15 percent more common in those who suffer from Down syndrome than in the remainder people. This may cause issues but not always in their language and speech but in their development of social skills. This is another reason that speech and language specialists are able to assist children suffering from Down syndrome.

What Can an Speech and Language Therapist Help?

Many will argue it is speech therapy that's the primary treatment for children suffering from Down syndrome. For cognitive development, children need vocabulary. The acquired language is used to help with thinking, reasoning and memory. Although these cognitive processes don't happen out loud, they still require words and language.

By using language and vocabulary children are better equipped to regulate their behavior. If you take a look at the "terrible 2s," most toddler outbursts are due to anger because they are unable to communicate what they'd like. Therapists for speech and language assist children with Down syndrome to communicate how they are feeling and what they would like or require. This can greatly improve their behavior and, in turn, helps with social interactions.

Parents will always be the ones who will be the primary therapists for children suffering from Down syndrome, as well as difficulties with speech and language and speech and language delays, since it is the daily interactions between families that provide the perfect environment for language. The speech and language therapy can assist parents in focusing on four key areas of comprehension such as grammar, vocabulary as well as reading, writing and signing.

Initial interactions will include you having your language and speech therapy therapist teaching you the most effective methods to apply at home. Much of it will be based on play. They'll be able to aid by using visual aids, such as flash cards. Many children who have Down syndrome learn the sign language to assist them in their communication throughout the beginning years, as their spoken communication skills grow.

If your child has hearing issues, an ear or nose and throat (ENT) specialist could recommend a small dosage of antibiotics or recommend hearing aids.

Now that we have looked at the various possible problems with speech and language you're probably eager to know how you can assist your child to get the most effective start to communication possible. The next chapters will cover the different therapies that are available, and what you can try at your home.

Chapter 11: Interaction Between A Child And A Parent

Parent-child interaction is also referred to by the name of parent-child interaction therapy (PCI or PCIT) and was created during the 70s. Dr. Sheila Eyberg developed PCI from three parenting strategies or developmental issues. This was Bowly's attachment theory researchand Baumrind's parenting techniques research, and Bandura's Social Learning theory. After more than 50 years of research advancements and positive results, PCI has now been modified to address a variety of childhood disorders, ranging including abuse and trauma as well as ASD and loss of hearing.

What is PCI?

The purpose for PCI treatment is to instruct parents how to communicate with their children in a way they can develop the desired behavior. To develop speech and language we've already observed the importance of parents being the primary caregivers. In this regard, therapists collaborate with parents to ensure they can enhance their emotional communication abilities and improve their positive interactions. This is usually done through live sessions. Therapists may film children and parents interacting, and use the footage to draw attention to learning opportunities. Other parents can watch their parents engage with children within a safe space (like their workplace) and then guide them employing an earpiece. In the wake of COVID crises, PCIT sessions have also successfully been held on the internet.

The format of the PCI session is different between children. The duration of each session may vary, but it's typical to attend only one session per week. In this class you will be provided with homework assignments and five-minute tasks that you can work on during the week. There are two major focuses of PCI which is child-directed interactions (which assists in improving the relationship between parents and children) as well as parent-directed interactions (when it is focused on behavior).

It is clear that PCI is a game changer in the field in the field of developmental child. However, evidence to support that it is effective in promoting language and speech development is still in the beginning stages. The most significant research was conducted on a sample of 18 children who had delayed development of their language along with their caregivers. The results were very positive, with a rise in the frequency of utterances and repetition.

Let's have a look at the PCI process, and particularly with one of the newest methods, the VERVE method of interaction with children. Keena Cummins has utilised PCI and other similar methods to create an "adult quiet, child-like watching technique that is based on videos to observe and self-reflection. The benefit of VERVE is Keena Cummins works as a speech and language therapy. Therefore, the approach focuses on communication and not the behavioral issues that children face.

There are five main components of VERVE

Video Parents are recorded as they interact with their children. Each session is 1 hour long. There are at a minimum, four three-minute sessions, each based on from the last session.

Endorse: Parents choose one important interaction skill and develop this one skill specifically. The skills for interaction could include the ability to name, repeat pausing or looking for eye contact, etc. If only one skill is in focus it is less confusing and the child is more at mastering this ability. Once the skill is mastery and mastered, the focus will be on developing another.

Respect: It is essential that parents look at their videos in order they can express their opinions, feelings and ideas about their child's growth.

Parents must feel respected and valued to be able to contribute ideas to improve their family's situation. The videos are an excellent way to observe the way they interact and to discover how they can improve their communication skills better. The videos also provide parents the chance to look back and look at the advancement their child is making.

Vitalise: Parents and the child can take part in this exciting and fulfilling experience. Parents can see how their skills are developing and the child develops more confidence when it comes to exploring and playing. Positive behavior is reduced and replaced by positive ones.

Eye contact The parents wait for their child to make eye contact prior to speaking. In this allows the child to listen to the words and then connect with reading the parents their lips and facial expressions. This can help improve their language skills.

Who can PCI help?

Be aware that therapy for parent-child interaction can assist parents with many different issues, including those that are related to behavioural issues. PCI is also a great option for a wide range of issues with language and speech, however, it is particularly effective for delays in speech development, ASD, delayed social skills , and hearing loss.

Speech delays: Parents are taught methods to improve their communication skills and not just during the therapy sessions. Parents can apply lessons learned and can be applied to all stages of a child's development. For children who have difficulty speaking the act of asking questions can cause anxiety and may contribute to their difficulty in understanding. PCI concentrates on expressing comments on the child's activities. Making comments and repeating actions during the play can encourage engagement. Parents are then taught to include words in the child's activities to broaden their vocabulary and grammar to create sentences.

ASD The most fascinating concerning PCI as well as ASD is that research has demonstrated that following the practice of PCI parents begin to look at their ASD child's issues differently and believe that they are not as difficult as they were prior to therapy. ASD children with problems with social interaction and/or speech and language difficulties are often faced with behavioural issues at some point during their lives due to their anger. PCI can help reduce the frequency of behavioural issues and meltdowns by around 85 percent in children aged 30 and 96 month. This type of therapy could be a catalyst for the development of self-esteem which could improve the development of language and speech.

Social skills that are not as developed: PCI originates from Bandura's social learning theory. It is therefore logical that this type of therapy is able to aid children with delayed social abilities. The concept lies on requirement to observe, model and imitating the behaviors, emotional reactions and attitudes of others. It's not because parents make the wrong social choices. We've also learned from the actions of others. PCI helps parents correct any issues with their own actions so that children are more positive role models for social situations.

Loss of hearing: PCI helps parents be more attentive to their child's needs, and teach parents how to be more responsive and emotionally accessible. The study looked at 18 children aged between the ages of 2 and 6 years old. They attended 16 sessions per week. Children who were treated with PCI therapy showed better behaviour as well as social skills, and also significant improvement in their communication skills.

PCI, PCIT and VERVE appear to be basic, yet they deliver impressive results. It's about shifting the focus away from the parent and letting the child take charge of the play. The goal is to reinforce positive behavior so that negative behaviors gradually fade away. It's a safe place for children, as well as offering a wealth of learning opportunities to parents. Research has been very limited, however the results are always positive. The techniques parents learn through PCI give a new outlook for achieving life-long benefits.

Chapter 12: Language As Well As Makaton To

Speech And Language Development

Before we get into the differences between Makaton and sign language Makaton and Makaton, let us put the myths that surround them to rest. Parents are concerned about the fact that learning sign language or Makaton can hinder the development of speech and language. They are concerned that children will get comfortable with signs and this can hinder them from learning to speak. The latest research shows that this is not the reality.

Research has proven how teaching kids alternative communications does not stop children from speaking but it can help them improve their ability to talk, regardless of whether the child is older or younger. In addition, it has been proven to boost cognitive abilities in children who do not have hearing loss or issues. Imagine signing your child; you're giving them an instrument to communicate prior to the normal stage of development in speech. For children who have speech and difficulties with language alternative communication allows them to communicate . This could encourage them to start speaking because of the positive experiences they've experienced with signing.

What is Sign Language?

The most important issue is what does it mean to be British Sign Language (BSL)? BSL is an officially recognized language which has been in use for over 250 years, since Thomas Braidwood founded the first deaf school in Scotland. The year 2003 was the time it was officially declared as an official language. similar to British English, it has its own grammar structure and regional dialects. British Sign Language is used by adults and children with hearing impairments. If a child is affected by hearing loss, the primary language will be BSL. They may also be able learn spoken English by using assistive listening devices. This is, when you think about it, is quite awesome because they'll be bilingual.

It is important to note that just like American as well as British English have their differences as are American as well as British Sign Language. Even between cities there will be minor differences and colloquialisms.

BSL is composed of a mixture of fingerspelling and signs. For instance, you can spell the word'sorry using your left hand in the middle of your chest, and then making circles in an anticlockwise direction. In order to spell words, make various forms using your fingers. Some are more simple because they resemble letters. For example, crossing two index fingers creates the letter "x". Even the less easy ones share a connection. An 's' is formed by putting your right baby finger with your left finger. It is possible to use your right index finger towards the tips of your fingers in the left hand (beginning through your thumb) for each vowel. Keep in mind when you speak left handed BSL the gestures are reversed. The british-sign.co.uk website is full of great sources to help you learners learn British Sign Language plus a fun game for spelling fingers.

What is Makaton?

In the 1970s In the 1970s, three Speech and Language Therapists invented Makaton as a language system comprised of symbols and signs. They were referred to as Margret Walker, Katherine Johnston and Tony Cornforth and this is significant as If you take the first two/three letters of their names in the beginning then you will have the word Makaton..

Certain signs are derived from BSL however the two systems can't be interchanged. The major distinction in Makaton in comparison to BSL can be seen in the way that Makaton is used in conjunction with speech, making it an aid to hearing children who need to develop their language. Once their language has grown sufficiently, they can not be using symbolism and signs.

Makaton makes use of symbols and signs, together with spoken words. For instance the sign for "where the hands are held with their palms open, facing upwards and putting hands in a downwards circle. The symbol that represents 'where' is the question mark. When dealing with symbols, it's crucial that the appropriate symbol is employed to provide the greatest clarity as possible, which is why there may be multiple symbols for a term. The triangular symbol is used of the verb "can," and 'a bottle of water is used to speak of a noun. Two signs are also used for the verb "eat" dependent on whether you're eating using your fingers or cuttinglery.

The best thing about Makaton is that it can be seen on TV. It is possible to watch "Something Special" on BBC and see how Mr. Tumble helps teach kids Makaton symbols and signs. Another favorite is 'CBeebies' Bedtime Stories'. This isn't exclusively for kids. There's a chance to see Makaton appearing in soap operas' storylines like "Eastenders" and "Emmerdale.".

Makaton is used today in more than 40 countries. As with the sign language, it is important to ensure that the resources you utilize are appropriate to what language the child will need assistance with. Therapists for speech or language should have lots of resources to help you, as well as the makaton.org website, particularly in case you're looking for assistance in languages other than English.

Does My Child Really Need BSL Or Makaton?

In reality, it's going to fall to your team of experts. Keep in mind it is true that BSL is the primary language spoken by the deaf community of the UK and Makaton is used to assist those children and have difficulty communicating. Both can result in incredible changes to a child's development and confidence, and there's absolutely nothing wrong with you and your kid watching a little of Mr. Tumble and learning some basic communication techniques.

Parents and Kids demonstrating Simple Makaton Signs You can Learn

We all know that books are more fascinating by having a few pictures. We've taken twenty of the most common and easy ways to begin with your kids. I'd like to take this opportunity to acknowledge all parents and kids from all over the world countries who contributed to this section of this book. They are all stars! !

Chapter 13: The Treatments You Can Try At Home

This is a huge chapter which I have packed with thoughts. These treatments can be utilized to treat the issues and delays we've been through. You may either choose to choose a specific therapy your speech and therapy therapist recommends or select what your child will like the most. Do not feel that you need to purchase all the latest gadgets and toys. There are plenty of ideas for items you could make use of that are already within your home.

Each of these treatments can be utilized for speaking and developing language. To help with speech, play back the words that they are unable to understand in a concise method to stimulate listening. For the language, the sky's the limit. Utilize these methods to expand on the language structure of "The toy is on the table/under the table/next table', or sequencing such as "First we'll... after that we'll' and, of course asking age-appropriate questions like 'What do would like to do with this toy Do you want to play with the toy?'.

Let's begin!

Aiding your child develop pre-verbal communication

It's not necessary to wait for the first words to begin helping them master these early skills of communication.

The "Means, Reasons and Opportunities model is based upon the research of Dr. Della Money in 1997:

What is the method by which children communicate. As we've seen, it could be verbal, like words and babbling, or non-verbal like gestures, pointing out or signs.

The reasons children have for communicating include expressing their desires, needs and emotions. There are some motivations that help to encourage the motivations. These could be their most loved toys, music or games. It is important to understand the motives and motivations for your child.

Opportunities: To help encourage the flow of communication, give them the greatest amount of opportunities. In order to do this, you'll often discover that you must look back. We as parents become very adept in anticipating the needs of our children. We can tell when they are hungry, thirsty , or exhausted before they even realize it. Due to this, we usually plan the things they require before they even ask for it. Our superpowers are not working since it means that they don't have the chance to express themselves. You'll always be eager to assist them however, if you are patient for a few minutes and you'll see that they are beginning to talk to you and tell them what they require or would like to know. There are many other methods to set up opportunities. For example, you could give the child an item paper and there is no crayon. Now you have the chance for your child to request crayons with their own methods. There is the possibility to incorporate language into the gestures, so you could say, "Oh you'd like an crayon?' or 'You are looking to color with an crayon?' would like a green, yellow or red crayon?'. You can give a yoghurt without spoon, offer crafting paper with no scissors and the list goes on. Place the toy your child is most fond of in a safe place, perhaps inside a transparent box to ensure that they'll require your assistance to retrieve the toy or play.

Reference Objects:

* Objects of Reference' (OOR) is the use of objects in a consistent manner to communicate. A reference object is any object that is regularly used to signify an item or activity, location or

the person. Understanding the real world is the initial stage in symbol development.

* objects can be used to represent events, activities or people, as well as locations.

* They may aid people in understanding and communicate about changes to their everyday routines. OOR can benefit children who suffer from visual impairments and hearing impairment. Social communication, or Autistic spectrum disorders (ASD) and/or Learning problems.

For introducing Objects of Reference, choose things and events the individual often participates in.

Find objects that can represent this event in a meaningful manner for the child.

* Before making a transition or performing something and demonstrating the object, demonstrate it and make use of simple language to explain to them what's happening.

Use the order in which your child's understanding of symbols develops and the stage of development your child is in: (real objects, miniature replicas of real objects pictures, line drawings writing, signs)

Things to keep in mind when selecting objects:

* Select real-life objects, like car keys that could be meaningful.

Smaller versions of items associated with an activity could be used, but they can occasionally be confusing for the child.

* objects of reference do not need to be a complete object, but can have shared characteristics, for example, the use of a cloth or towel to symbolize taking bathing.

Take into consideration the child's sensory needs when they have a low tolerance for a particular type of texture it won't be an ideal object for to use as a reference.

* You might be interested in determining if the item is able to be repaired if it is damaged or destroyed.

It is important to encourage your child to keep the object in their hands on their way to the event or until they recognize the person or person (bear be aware that it could take time for your child to get used to it).

* Consistency is the most important thing! Therefore, use identical objects, explain it the same way and employ the same language to describe the event or person etc.

Make use of the objects to teach concepts to children, and children can use references to ask questions.

* Safety is a further aspect to consider - the headphones can be good as an OCR, but the wire could pose a risk. Consider also whether the product be cleaned easily if needed? Does it break, or cause injury when they try to explore it using their mouths, or is there a chance of choking or swallowing the object?

* It can take some time for children to become adjusted to OOR.

Strategies for treating Developmental Learning Disorder (DLD)

Make sure you get your child's attention and shout their name prior to speaking to them or give them instructions.

Make use of visual cues, such as pictures, gestures or even acting out things.

* Use a simple and recurrent language.

* Provide instructions in smaller portions.

* Check for understanding. For instance, following an instruction ask your child what do you want your mommy to do? Repetition the instructions if necessary. Only give one instruction at one moment. For example, go get

you book. Go get your pencil. Relax and complete your homework. Instead of saying go to the library, get your pencil, then, sit down at the table to finish your assignment.

* Allow more time for your child to process what you've directed them to do.

* Do not be afraid to give plenty of praise and positive words.

Encourage the child's use of non-verbal communication to communicate and communicate their message. Facilitate communication by allowing their non-verbal communication.

Strategies to combat Selective Mutism school or outside of the home

* Accept non-verbal communication

* Reducing or removing pressure to talk

Participate with the child in activities in the classroom that don't require them to speak. For example, ask them to give out books/pens/pencils/paper to their peers. Request the child to help to gather things from others, but do not just pick them out, as the attention of others isn't something a child is likely to like.

Incorporate this child into the adult group led by a non-verbal child activities.

* Praise every child for their excellent communication.

If you can, choose one primary person spend time one-on-one with the child to help build confidence and build rapport. As time passes, the child might start to whisper , then perhaps talk, but keep in mind that if the child is having difficulty, it's because they really can't speak/talk therefore patience is crucial.

Stuttering/Stammering Strategies:

* Balance questions and comments while interacting with your child.

* Ask questions when feasible.

* Ensure that the child who struggles with speech is given equal opportunity both at home and in the classroom, to speak the same way as their peers or siblings.

* Request their peers and siblings not to speak on their behalf.

* Don't complete the sentence of your child if they get into a struggle.

* Do not try to try to guess what they're trying to convey, ...just allow them to speak to reassure yourself that you're paying attention.

Make sure your child knows you're listening. Get at their level and keep eye contact.

* Allow them time to finish their speech - refrain from interrupting.

* Reduce your speech speed Make sure to take a few pausing when speaking. This helps your child feel less stressed when they talk.

Recognize your child's feelings regarding their stammering. Calmly tell them, 'I see you're angry, and assure them that you're listening.

If your child gives up in speaking, let them know about the stammering e.g. gradually say, "I can understand that the word was difficult to pronounce'.

• Tell the other adults in the life of your child this suggestion so that everyone reacts in exactly the same way.

The importance of playing and Social Communication

After looking into PCI, Lego therapy, and intense interactions, you've likely realized the value of playing, and not only for children. Play can be a huge benefit for parents as well as any other members of the household. We will examine two additional therapies that are based on play, one is Lego Therapy and the second is a collection of Interaction therapies.

In the meantime, we will look at some incredible play concepts for various age groups, disabilities, delays and levels.

Lego Therapy

An interesting information for you There exist 62 sets of Lego for each person on the planet!

Parents have a love/hate relationship Lego. Cleaning up all these little bricks is an issue and they manage to get them to the most difficult-to-reach places such as under the couch! It's difficult to find anyone who hasn't shouted when they stepped on one of the pieces of Lego. However when we get together with our kids and let their imaginations run wild for a while, Lego is actually quite enjoyable and helps to relieve the stress that we have built up.

The act of playing with Lego is the same as playing with Lego and has the same relaxing impact on children. It also helps children learn to conquer the challenges of frustration, patience, and focus. We're just beginning to explore the benefits in the development of speech and language! It took a surprising 70 years to get this loved toy to be used as a therapy tool thanks to Dr. LeGoff. A clinical neuropsychologist observed that children suffering from ASD and other social difficulties were attracted towards playing Lego. If Lego games are structured and children are encouraged to play, they can develop the social skills of a variety of children.

LeGoff's study found that children between the six and sixteen experienced significant improvements in three areas of social competency following Lego therapy. They showed improvement in the beginning of social interaction with peers and the ability to keep relationships, in addition to the reduction of stereotyped behaviours. A few years later, LeGoff conducted a second study which showed Lego therapy can also enhance collaborative problem solving tasks, task focus, taking turns and sharing.

What is the best way to use Lego Therapy Work?

Lego therapy is typically used with children who are between 5 and 17. The best part is that the difficulty level can be easily adapted to any age group , and for expressive and receptive issues with language as well as social communication issues. In general, there are groups comprising three children and one adult. Every child is assigned one of the roles listed below such as the Engineer (or the Architect) as well as the Supplier as well as the Construction. Let's look more closely at each one of the roles:

The The Engineer's task is to ensure that the supplier has the correct bricks and the Builder will be able to acquire the entire set. They will outline the steps needed by the Builder to build the model and will be able to answer any construction-related questions that might arise. When the model is complete they will verify whether it's correct.

A Supplier is required to arrange the various bricks required. They should follow the instructions from the Engineer, and then give the appropriate bricks to Builder. They may also inquire about things that require clarification. The toughest part for the Supplier is being patient between turns.

The Builder When they have received all the bricks they need from the supplier and have listened to the instructions of the Engineer to put models together. builder can inquire of the Engineer questions, and then they'll have to figure out how to stay on the line between turns.

The adult participant must be seated at a distance and assume the role of facilitator and not leader. If an adult assumes the role of Engineer or the Supplier or Builder, it can lead to an inability to communicate with the group. The adult will be there to give suggestions and only intervene when they feel the group is getting frustrated in the game. To provide suggestions for the group, the adult may make use of things like an image-based checklist or name guide to help with Lego names. Lego names. It is important to praise the kids for the tasks they are able to successfully complete.

What can children gain What can children gain from Lego Therapy?

Personally, I like the idea of children playing with a plaything that is non-discriminating, gender neutral and enjoyable for everyone. Every play-based space is going aid in removing the anxiety that may arise when meeting new people. And for children older than 10 it could help eliminate the stigma that is associated with the traditional methods of therapy.

Lego therapy is a great way for children develop the ability to move and develop memory skills. It helps them focus on planning and sequencing, as well as listening and asking questions. Children need to concentrate on visual images to produce something tangible. So, in addition to visual perception, you will notice a huge confidence boost after the team has completed its mission. The encouragement may cause youngsters to desire new things in different social settings. For their language skills they can improve their vocabulary and the descriptive language and their positional.

Who is the person who can Lego Therapy help?

Lego therapy is a great option for every child struggling with language and speech development. The roles of the Engineer, Builder and Supplier help to reinforce the essential vocabulary and language concepts that could be applied into other areas of learning and daily life. For instance, the positional language can help children comprehend concepts such as "on top of" or 'next to', as well as "beside". Descriptive language expands their vocabulary of adjectives and adjectival terms. Dependent on their age, they also practice the concepts of sequentiality, like "first" and "next'. If you are able to imagine all the things you can construct with Lego and other Lego products, you will be able to appreciate the potential of learning languages.

In particular, Lego therapy is the ideal solution for children with difficulty with speech or language caused by social situations. This can be due to speech stuttering, selective mutism, anxiety, or even autism. The removal of children from the bustling class and working in smaller groups takes a great deal of stress from the child. They can feel safe , and since the activities are child-led instead of adult-led, they can be more confident in executing their abilities and communicating. As children's confidence starts to build, they'll be capable of transferring the vast array of abilities they've acquired via Lego therapy into other areas such as the playground or even smaller groups in the classroom.

A better question is the following: Who is Lego therapy not appropriate for? It's unlikely you'll see the full benefit of Lego therapy for children with behavioural problems that are not related to problems with speech or language. It might not be suitable for children suffering from ADHD (attention deficiency hyperactivity disorder). The issue here is that kids with these kinds of issues could be disruptive to the class or playing a specific part. Consider inviting your two most cherished acquaintances to dinner alongside the queen of England The one of them is bound be the star of the evening regardless of whether she intends at it or not! Because each of these three roles requires listening, speaking and turning it is recommended to form an organization that is, to a certain extent, like.

Another wonderful aspect of Lego therapy are the number of free sources that are available. My personal favorite is twinkl.co.uk. It is a site where you can search for "building blocks therapy'. Print adult guidance, language positional cards Key word cards brick-building cards, and much more at no cost. There are a lot of instructional videos available on YouTube which can assist you get more comfortable in being the facilitator prior to you introduce Lego therapy for your kid. It is possible to have a regular "Lego party" or invite your kid's classmates to come along and play in the event that you think it's the right thing to do or you might have siblings who would like to join in.

Interactive Interaction

The name for this kind of therapy may sound intimidating, but it can be a lot of fun. As with PCI intensive interaction, it is an approach to the development of communication partners so that they can achieve greater results. Let's begin from the beginning.

David Hewett was a principal of a school for special needs close to London. In the 1980s, there was not as much information about the special education that it is now. There were no tools for teaching for people with significant difficulties communicating. Hewett would like to teach his pupils , but he soon discovered that when he and his staff were unable to break down the initial barriers and get to know their students, the learning process could be unproductive. Studies on interactions that began in the infant years, coupled with meticulous trial and error as well as paying attention to how students were reacting in a way, led to a lot of interactions.

The method focuses on those crucial first interactions, that it initially known as "augmented mothering". It takes the complicated interactions between toddlers and babies in the early two years of life and applies the same interactions to children with more serious communication, language, and speech issues. Studies have shown positive effects for children and adults, hence its name changed from "intensive interaction'.

What are the effects of intensive interaction?

A few people get shocked initially. The partner in communication (most probably you) is required to modify behavior which would otherwise seem normal. It is ironic that the communication between parents and their baby is perhaps the most natural communication there is. Consider the times when your baby was just a baby. here are a few essentials of first communication stage:

* Learning to utilize and comprehend eye contact

* Use facial expressions and reading

• Learning to utilize and comprehend physical contact

* Learning to utilize and comprehend non-verbal communication

The concept of intensive interaction is taken and extends them including things such as:

* Helping to develop concentration and focus

* Reversing their behaviours and interactions

* Copying sequences from the activities of other people

* Sharing appreciation and your personal space

* Learning to manage levels of excitement

Most importantly, engaging in a lot of conversation involves taking an extra step and learning how to be a good friend in your home with your kid. Without fault of our own it is the case that time has a way of taking over us. Babies even however much we love they really don't have to do well, but we can be awestruck and in amazement. We are able to be content in the slow lane for a few minutes. Interactions that are intense remind us that speed is reserved for special events and is not something to be enjoyed!

What kind of intensive interaction is required from the Communicator?

There are a lot of things that speech and language therapists can impart to you. But, prior to you can do that, I believe it's crucial to are in the proper mental state of mind. In intense interactions it is essential to focus on the moment, removing the worries of your daily life and giving all of your attention on your little one. It is essential to be ready to enjoy yourself. The intense interaction method could then be an integral part of your daily routine. It could be in routine activities, at periods of quiet or when your child is showing indications of wanting to become social. It is also possible to set aside the time each day to get to know each other better.

A significant change is in your voice tone or your eye contact, as well as other body language. These modifications will allow you to not be as intimidating so please don't interpret it the wrong way. As an mother, I'd not want to think of my behavior as intimidating and being a speech and language therapy therapist I understand that standing up when talking to children is often like you're in a position of dominance over them. If you can get to their level, by sitting on the ground with them and then suddenly they will be more at ease.

It is also possible to learn to detect the subtle signals that your child communicates to you. You might notice that your child is avoiding you when they want to take a break from the task or may exhibit an unusual behavior that helps calm them down. A psychologist observed that children would touch his or her hands using their thumb. If the therapist began to press their thumbs into the palm of the child and the child reacted by rubbing the palm of the therapist by using their own thumb. This was the very first stage of their interactions in the beginning, which grew so fast that eventually the child began to be able to sing along with the therapist.

Like PCI as with PCI, it is the child who must be the one to decide on activities as the adult is present to mostly comment and react. It is also important for a rhythm and repetition to ensure that you keep the attention of your child and help them to anticipate what is going to occur in the next.

Possible outcomes from Intensive Interaction Therapy

Different studies have been conducted on children in various ages, and all of which have shown positive outcomes. The research has shown that intensive interaction with others increases social engagement as well as the initiation process, as well as more eye contact, smiling and looking up at faces. A few studies have revealed kids are less accepting when it comes to contact with physical. There has also been improvement in the way they speak. While each child is bound react differently, parents will concur that children generally feel happier after an intensive time of interactions.

Who Can Benefit from Intensive Interaction?

David Hewett, along with his colleague Melanie Nind, has stated that intensive interactions are the most beneficial for people with S/PMLD . This includes those who have extremely or profound and multi learning disabilities, particularly those who are either non-verbal or preverbal. This is certainly true for children with extreme autism, or Down syndrome. It's dependent on the specialists on your team and your child's needs in regards to whether or not they feel that intense interaction with your child will benefit them.

One thing to keep in mind is that intensive interactions require professional training. Contrary to Lego therapy and other similar activities, it's not something that you download resources and start at home. While you're waiting to meet the speech and language specialist you are able to try some of the basics we've looked at including things like committing each day to sit on the ground with your child. Allow them to pick the play game and then you watch and observe.

What is social interaction? Interaction

Keep in mind that we are discussing a range of issues for children in relation to interactions with others. Your child may be appearing awkward in social settings or perhaps the stress is too much that they are unable to communicate in social settings. It is crucial to keep in mind to remember that having a language or language disorder does not guarantee that this will happen. There are many children who suffer from problems with speech or language are likely to have difficulties in social situations. However children who speak fairly well for their age, however they still have to improve their social interaction. This is known as "pragmatics or 'pragmatics'. This is the case when children don't grasp the social norms that are required to effectively communicate with family, friends and teachers. Here are a few examples of the acceptable rules for social communication:

* Utilizing the appropriate level of English to serve various purposes, such as greeting people or to request things, or to inform

* Adjusting or changing the language level based on the person you're talking to and in different settings and knowing how much information you can provide to a listener

* Respecting the other participants having a turn in conversations

* Introduce a topic while staying on the topic

* Use the appropriate body expressions and facial expressions and eye contact

There's no way you'll be witnessing your child of two or three years grasp the art of media. They'll open their mouths and speak in a way that makes you wish the ground take you away. Social communication can be learned over a long period of time and, even after that, not everyone is able to say they have it perfectly every time, especially when it comes to cultural distinctions.

The speech and language therapy therapist could help children struggling with social interactions, even if an issue with speech or language isn't yet diagnosed. The focus will be placed on play-based therapy and strategies can be used at home.

What exactly is Early Interaction?

We've discussed early interactions in various ways. It's about the ways you can play with newborns and infants to help them develop the very first essential steps of communication. Early interactions encompass all the sounds that babies hear and the expressions at people's faces, and the various gestures. Listening to Mum and Dad's voices from in the early years will aid in the development of speech This begins long even before the baby is born - they're able to hear every thing that happens out in the world outside of the comfort of their baby's womb.

There is a benefit to newborns. We're so impressed by them that it's simple to observe them for a while despite the fact that they're not doing a lot of amount. This is the ideal moment to start early interactions. Infants can see around 20-30cm away, so ensure that you're close enough to allow them to observe your face as well as the various expressions you use. Soon they begin to be able to focus their eyes on different objects. At that point you can begin showing them various toys and household objects, and telling the story behind them. This will also motivate children to begin making a move and try to grasp objects.

Babies must be loved and held. They need to feel the warmth and love of your arms. This is important to keep them safe and also to build their self-confidence and self-esteem. Do not worry about coddling them and instilling independence. There is plenty of time to be all by them while they're sleeping. They'll have only very short attention spans when they reach this point, and there's no need to be overly attentive at this time.

When your baby is just a couple of months old, they'll begin to love listening to your singing and reciting rhymes. Like every interaction with children whatever age they are, you must to be completely engaged and at ease. Do not feel that you have to always be at the center of attention. The first moments of your interactions must be a bit more casual even if it's just to take in their beautiful smile and a few laughter.

Children who have delayed early interaction skills have trouble sharing toys with classmates or their siblings at nursery. Some children are very shy and find It difficult to speak in the nursery and participate playing activities with their friends. Certain children are unable to engage in conversation like, for instance, the child who is four would like to, they might not be able to inquire whether they are allowed to participate in an activity that their friends are taking part in. They might stand at a distance , and observe their friends playing, but they are not sufficiently confident to participate. This is why the support of an adult is needed to help children interact to their friends and gain confidence when communicating.

Sometimes, a delay in communication can be the most significant barrier faced by children, and they are often isolated when the proper support isn't provided. Your speech therapist is competent to guide you to play with the communication strategies at the home of your child in which you will involve your children's siblings, cousins , or other children of friends as well as advise that the child's nursery put plans in the place to assist your child improve in engaging with peers and adults in their surroundings.

Tips to Help You Practice Play at Home

This section we're going to review some of the top games, books and toys that can help develop speech and language skills as also early interaction as well as social interaction.

Books

It's amazing that there are so many amazing books available for kids. The most popular books to help boost the language, speech and rhymes include:

* "The Hungry Caterpillar"
* "The Busy Spider' Busy Spider'
* "Brown Bear, Brown Bear, What do you see What do you see?
* The "Chicka" set
* 'Go, Dog, Go'
* "The Rainbow Fish'
* 'Goodnight Moon'
* "Where the Wild Things Are'
* "We're Going to Bear Hunt'
* "Spot the Dog'

Personally, I am a fan of every single one of Julia Donaldson books, particularly the Songbirds collection, which was developed by Oxford Owl and which focus on phonetics. It is also a good idea to keep your eyes open for tactile books for your child that stimulate participation. If you're in search of additional guidance on social interactions, make or find your own social stories which I have discussed in depth in my book on Understanding Autism, Potty Training and Personal Care Let your child perform basic hygiene tasks like getting haircuts, brushing their teeth cleaning hands and bathing, and more! Click here to buy the book if interested. http://mybook.to/UAPTpersonalcare

Toys

There are a few items that almost every child owns, apart from the Lego set! These include usually figures, dolls and animal farm sets. They are great for the role-playing process. Role-playing lets children act out scenarios that could make them feel anxious or uncomfortable. It helps them prepare for future events and, naturally there's a broad variety of vocabulary and concepts that are able to be learned. Shape sorters can be useful for concentration and prepositions. Play-Doh, similar to Lego is a toy with unlimited possibilities for vocabulary. If you can, purchase gender neutral toys. There's no reason girls to have specific toys, and girls to play with other.

Games to take turns

There are plenty of exciting board games to teach kids how important it is to take turns. "Candy Land," "Hi Ho Cherry-O' and "Let's fish' appropriate for children aged 3 and over. For children who are beginning to master this social skill earlier, it is best to avoid board games since they contain tiny parts that can be risky. Use routine activities to teach your child how to play. It could be something easy like mixing cake batter, in which you get to take turns and then they get the chance to take their turn. You can also employ stickers, where the children select one to stick on their drawings, then you.

Jenga is great for everyone in terms of safety , but in terms of skill it's not as great. But, older kids will delight in removing bricks while younger kids can rotate to put the bricks over each the other.

Games to practice eye Contact

"Pass the Smile" is a fun game that is played by just two players but it's best played playing in groups. You sit in a circle, and pick a facial expression. smiles are the most popular but you could also choose to pass the wink for instance. One person, wearing an unassuming facial expression turns to the person in front of them and smiles. The next person smiles, then turns at the person next to them and hands it over. You can also play the game using the ball.

Two people can play the mirror match game. You sit in front of each the other (or place yourself in a stand) and one of you is chosen to be the mirror. They must copy every move the mirror does. It is possible to start by doing simple movements like facial expressions, then progress to movement of the legs and arms. Puppets can also create a magical impact on children and draw their interest. When the puppets whisper into your ear' children are drawn to your face.

How to Create an Imaginative Play with a Budget

Wouldn't it be nice to have the money to buy all the top games and books for your children and grandchildren! The reality isn't always like that however this isn't a problem. Here are four suggestions for how you can try with your kids with items are already in your kitchen cupboards.

* homemade bubbles 1 , 1/2 cup of water 1 cup of washing liquid two teaspoons sugar. You can make use of an old coat hanger wire to create the bubble wand.

Playdough: 2 cups flour 1/4 cup salt 4 tablespoons of cream tartar 2 cups of lukewarm water 2 tablespoons of coconut or vegetable oil. Mix all the ingredients together in a pan at a low temperature until it becomes a smooth ball. Allow it to cool down for a few minutes and then divide in smaller pieces, then knead some with food coloring. Place the mixture in Ziploc bags, and it should last for a couple of months.

- Social Stories: In the event that you are unable to find a story to print then you can create yourself stories. Photograph your child or download photos. You could fold the paper, write on it and draw images by hand if you do not have an printer. Your child can colour your drawings.

* Puppets: Does anyone not have a couple of bizarre socks, which the washer appears to have consumed? You can take all of the socks and draw characters on them. You can cut felt shapes and stick them on pipe cleaners or whatever else you might have in your crafting box. Should your toddler is in the process of putting things into their mouths, take care to make sure that nothing could be pulled out of the puppets.

Vocabulary Building Using Food

It will also assist those with a dietary problem to explore a wide range of food.

Prepare for massive quantities of fun. There will be some cleaning up afterward, but the mess of food play is definitely worth it. Make sure you have a tray to fill it with food items. You can make use of things like juice, milk and tomato sauce, mashed up bananas mousse, yoghurt, you know what you can use it for. If you're looking to make the mess to a minimum, consider dry foods such as cereals flour, sugar and cold cooked pasta, or rice. Put small toys (no risk of choking) within the food items and then take turns finding the toys.

If you're using liquids, then use the liquid inside the tray to create handprint images. You can also use the dried food along with PVC glue to create pictures and the pasta that has been cooked are able to be tied onto strings.

The most important thing is the time you've set aside for your child, allowing them to enjoy and play. There is no need for expensive toys as they aren't role models but you are! Making time to play with your child on a regular basis is crucial to their learning and confidence.

Strategy for Speech and Sound Development

In addition to the time you spend each day playing with your child it is also possible to employ the following strategies for developing speech sounds during the course of your day. This means that you should take advantage of your day-to-day activities to focus on certain sounds that your child is struggling with.

One thing I would suggest at this stage is to not keep correcting your child whenever they make mistakes in their speech or a sound, but instead concentrate on the method you correct them.

The aim is to increase their confidence as high as is possible. To do this, attempt in rephrasing words using the correct pronunciation, instead of using phrases like 'No do not say it like that, just say it this way.'

Auditory Bombardment

The year 1983 was when Hodson as well as Paden developed the practice of auditory bombardment therapy that is commonly utilized in conjunction with games in sessions of speech therapy and language. It is used, for instance at the beginning and the final stages in the course. The child is exposed to various examples of the phonological targets. Imagine that you're at the kitchen table together. you can repeat all the items you notice that begin with the sound you want to target"s/":'saucepan spoon' sausage,'sink' and on. Keep in mind that this is an exercise to listen, and it is important to practice the words but don't ask your child to speak the words.

It is interesting to note that the importance and advantages of bombardment with sound can be observed in studies of the cross-linguistic acquisition of phonological sounds. English children are more likely to develop the sound /v/ later during their development since it is not a standard phoneme in English language. When it comes to French kids, it is more likely that they develop the sound earlier because that they hear it often.

It's important to note that Hodson is now using the term "focused auditory stimulation' in reference to the somewhat aggressive interpretation of the word "bombardment'.

Rhyme/Rhythm

One thing that virtually every culture shares can be the usage of rhythm and rhyme in a variety of ways, not just to teach however, but as a method of passing on customs. A rhythmic structure and rhyme aid children as well as adults to recall and repeat words. There are also connections between the capacity to acquire the language of a child and musical skills. Musicians are able to understand and make particular sounds and patterns of sound. This is why when you incorporate music into the rhythm and rhyme, you'll be able to help your child develop.

I'm the first to admit that breaking into song during mid-day may be something a bit Disney-like, however, there are rhymes you can use throughout the day. These, when repeated, can make your kid want to join in.

(To the same tune as 'Happy Birthday To You')

Bonjour to everyone!

Hello to all!

Good morning dear child's name

Bonjour to everyone!

Clean up, clean up

Everyone, let's get it cleaned up

Clean up, clean up

Everyone is welcome!

(To similar tune to "Here We Go Round the Mulberry Bush')

This is how we wear our shirt

Don't forget to put on our shirt

Don't forget to put on our shirt

This is how we dress when we don our shirts.

It's early in the morning.

And, of course, don't ignore the old nursery rhymes we were taught when we were children. The study found that if children know at minimum eight nursery rhymes before they turn four, they'll be among the top in spelling and reading within their school. It's true that this is applicable to children of atypical age - however it is a good reminder of how important these classics from the past.

Utilizing rhymes or similar sound is a method that we employ with children who have difficulty making some sounds, but they do not realize they're making mistakes while speaking. For instance, a four year old child may be reducing sounds from clusters and Instead of using 'Sun' "Soup" and "Sock" the child is saying "Dun", "Doup," and "Dock". At home, you can try during your normal routines and dedicated playtime with your child to find words/items/activities that begin with the /s/ sound.

While out and about or shopping, search for things that start with the sound /s/. It is important to emphasize the /s/ sound at the beginning of every word and then repeat the word at least two times. For example: 'soup', 'seat', 'six', 'sad', 'salad', 'salt', 'same', 'sand', 'send' etc.

Look at the words that rhyme, and see how your child perceives the differences. Can they create rhyme-related words? For instance, if the sound you are aiming for will be /t/ then you can show images of things that start with the sound /t/ ('tea' ('two'), 'top tap') and also have images that begin with sound /ksound ('key", 'coo cop "', "cap'). Set the images ('tea'/'key') in front of your child. If you talk about one of the phrases ('Tea'), make sure that your child is not able to see your mouth. Does your child recognize the correct word simply through listening? If not, let them hear your voice when you speak the word.

The speech therapist will teach you and demonstrate this in the clinic if they believe this is suitable to your child. You will be provided with materials related to your desired sound that you can practice at home between the next time you visit.

Syllable Clapping

It is something that adults do not often think about but it is crucial for children to to understand what words look like as well as the various sounds contained within their structure. It is beneficial to teach children who have difficulty understanding the sounds in words. With practice, the aim is for them to make up the sounds missing by substituting any and then finally, the right sound.

If you're in need of to refresh your memory for a quick refresh, here's a short sentence that includes the syllable claps:

Instead of clapping your hands together it is also possible to clap one hand over the other, or tap the table. Some teachers at schools place their hands under their chins and each time their chin touches their hands the syllable is said to be. This is a great strategy for children who are unable to differentiate between syllables using making a clap. It may feel a awkward doing this, but I'm sure you're already trying it!

Encourage Listening Skills

We've previously discussed that listening is important, and your child is learning from your excellent model. In terms of listening strategies There are plenty of games to help your child engage in activities that require listening including "Simon Says," "Mother May I?' or "Red Light Green Light'.

Listening walks are the perfect way to encourage children to pay attention to the sounds we ignore. If you take the walk, stop for an instant while you close your eyes. while you're together, think about the sounds that you hear.

The television can be your greatest partner or biggest foe. There are plenty of excellent programs developed to promote education. If you want to make use of the television as a tool is to spend time with your child watching television and discuss what you are watching. Also, you should spend time with your family without the TV on to minimize the noise that your baby is exposed to.

Developing Speech Sounds Awareness

A child should acquire the ability to comprehend and listen to the sounds of rhyme, words, and syllables. This is essential to develop speech. Try these strategies to assist your child to improve their sound awareness

* Syllable clapping

Sound and Rhyme

* Sorting objects according to the sound that they first make (all objects beginning in the sound of /b/, such as "bottle," "bricks," and 'bat')

* Copying sounds The child should be the teacher, asking questions and then ask adults to duplicate the sounds. You will definitely make mistakes and your child will need to help you pronounce the correct words. This will aid in the child's learning process, and it's fun to watch Mommy and Daddy make mistakes! !

To assist children in identifying which sounds are similar or different, we employ basic pairs. It is crucial to figure the cause of your child's problems and whether they relate with their hearing. Does your child really be able to hear the sound they cannot recognize? Play a few games to find out. The speech therapist can examine your child in the smallest pairs, then show strategies and offer materials to help you practice at home.

Try the following to see if they be able to hear. Put one of the pictures before your child. Have an article that is paper, or even your palm on your lips. The goal is to ensure that your child is using only his or her listening abilities. Use just one sentence, e.g. "Tea. If your child selects the correct picture, tell them"Good listening. Then say 'Key. If they do are able to do it again you can praise them, then repeat "Key" again. If they are successful then that's great. If they say the word 'Tea', it means they thought you'd use the word "Tea" because you've just declared "Key". This is a bit similar to tricking your child, this is to ensure that they are capable of hearing what you're saying.

Chapter 14: The Understanding Of

Articulation And Phonological Disorder

It's essential to know the articulation or phonological disorders as this will help in the process of rehabilitation. It is important to remember that children of a young age will naturally have issues when learning to speak. However, as they get older they will be in a position to overcome these difficulties and articulate correctly.

If your child's speaking doesn't improve with age There must be something that is fundamentally wrong. If you've noticed difficulties with your child's speech it is important to determine the root cause so that you to address the issue effectively.

What causes speech problems?

Speech issues are disorders that are defined by the inability of a person to correctly pronounce words and to express himself. It's typically caused by an inefficient function of brain. It's a type of learning disability that may hinder the progress of a child's education.

What are the reasons for difficulties with speech?

There are a variety of causes of speech disorders. The majority of them are serious conditions that developed into speech disorders. Here are a few disorders that can cause speech disorders:

* Autism or Autism Spectrum Disorder (ASD)

It is a disorder of development where a child is experiencing an insufficient development of his language skills, social skills and behaviour. Watch your child closely and observe how they interact with others. Does he have trouble interacting with other children his age? Does he struggle to communicate? Does he seem to be isolated from his peers? If you said "Yes" to any of these questions then you must seek out a professional to determine whether your child is indeed suffering from ASD.

* Apraxia

This is also referred to also as Childhood Apraxia of Speech (CAS) It is characterised by the child's inability to speak the word, due to the fact that the muscles and the brain aren't in sync with one another. With this disorder of speech motors, your child might have difficulty in articulating long syllables and might tend to reduce or skip syllables challenging to pronounce. He is able to pronounce the words however he is unable to articulate it well. One example is when the speaker says "bana" in place of "banana" or "flor" instead of "flower".

* Intellectual disability

The disability is characterised by mental impedance. It is a sign that the problem with speech occurs because the child is experiencing delays in development throughout his life. It is natural that his development is slower than children older than him, and this is the reason he can't communicate effectively. The most important aspect of mental impairment can be that the kid is unable to grasp simple instructions and is prone to low memory.

* Neurological disorders

These are diseases that affect nerves and the brain, including muscular dystrophy, cerebral palsy and other brain diseases. These conditions can all cause problems with articulation, and can cause problems with phonology. Consult an expert in neurology if you suspect that your child suffers from this disorder. It can be a result of an accident, brain injuries or trauma, and sometimes, even severe shock.

* Auditory Processing Disorder (APD)

It is the capacity that the Central Nervous System (CNS) to process auditory signals. There are a variety of conditions that affect the process, including Attention Deficit Hyperactivity Disorder (ADHD) as well as autism and environmental circumstances (noisy environments). There are instances where the hearing organs fail which means they are not sending the correct signals to the brain.

The CNS is the brain that processes all signals sent through the various areas of the body. when the signals from nerves are not correctly interpreted, speaking and articulation may be difficult to achieve. The brain can also misinterpret how words sound meaning that the person will not be able speak the words correctly.

* Selective Mutism

This is a condition where children remain still in certain situations. In this case, the child is able to choose when to not speak. A good instance is when a child who is scared of his father, remains in silence when his father is near him. Another instance is when a child does not speak at school, due to fear of making a grammar mistake and being disregarded.

* Hearing loss

It is possible that you are unaware of it , but your child might not be hearing, which is the reason he isn't able to speak. Even when the time comes talk, it's difficult to understand. It is important to establish that your child isn't deaf prior to addressing the speech issues. An easy hearing test should suffice.

The steps to take for the easy hearing test:

1. Your child should be seated in the middle of a room.

2. Tell him to close his eyes.

3. Make two coins and place yourself on the other side of him, while staying a good distance from him.

4. Place the coins in your fingers, then click them against one another.

5. Keep clicking and ask him for the location of your computer.

6. Go to the right side and then click the coins once more.

7. Let him identify your location.

8. Take a look to the left and click the coins again.

9. Let him identify your position.

10. If he is not suffering from a hearing problem the person will be able to recognize every position you take.

11. If he does not perform the task, look at the ear responsible for the error and record your observations.

12. It is recommended to speak with your Eye Ear Nose and Throat (EENT) specialist in the event that you suspect he has a hearing problem. The EENT will commence treatment after the reason for the loss of hearing is identified.

13. If your child is not showing indications of hearing loss then you are able to follow the guidelines in this guide.

* Defects in speech organs

There could also be problems on his palate or vocal chords. It is recommended to consult with your physician to rule out aural and oral issues prior to beginning the exercises you are doing for your therapy. They will conduct an physical examination of the oral cavity and look the vocal cord for injury or palate damage.

After you've identified the root of your child's speech issues You can then begin to restore his speech . You can also use strategies to help him improve his pronunciation and Phonology.

Conclusion

As I've mentioned many times that listening skills are the foundation of all other language skills that your child has to develop to become a proficient language user. Being a proficient language user will allow your child to excel in social, academic and workplace settings.

As your child's skills in listening improve, they'll be more "tuned" to new words and grammar. If they spot new patterns, they'll be able to apply these within their language. This will enhance all aspects of communication, both expressively as well as openly.

Language skills that are good for children help them to be more successful in school. Language skills that are good for children help them improve their reading skills. The skills of a good language teacher help children communicate their needs, wants thoughts, ideas, data and feelings with greater ease.

Effective communication skills can aid your child in developing more positive relationships with adults and other peers. Improved relationships can boost your child's self-esteem as well as self-esteem. Effective communication skills can enable children to be leaders.

Communication skills that are effective aid children in becoming more confident.

It all begins with listening.

The book focuses specifically improving listening comprehension, however there's a different kind of listening was not much discussed however, it doesn't mean it's less essential. It's called social listening.

Social listening is the act of paying attention to what the individual speaker communicating via a range of actions, such as the tone of voice and body language. These actions or signals enable your child to identify a social situation and respond appropriately. This kind of social listening is just as crucial to listening skills.

For instance, if we're speaking to one of our friends and they're constantly checking their watches There's a good possibility of having to go away, but you don't want to come across as rude. A skilled speaker will recognize this and figure out a way to stop the conversation so that the person is able to focus on the task at hand.

A lot of times, children notice social cues. If your child is among those who don't, a bit of explaining and modeling can be a huge help in enhancing these abilities.

Another kind of hearing that parents are typically worried about too. Your children should adhere to your guidelines and adhere to your standards or perform the things you tell to do. This is a completely different style of listening, and is not the focus of this book. All I'll say is Good Luck!

It's clear, there are a myriad of ways to help your child improve their listening abilities. I'm sure that you will create more options than I did. The most important thing is to have fun and help your child especially when they're struggling.

Imagine what it would be to be like as a kid suffering from difficulty processing language. They can hear you, but they aren't able to figure out what they need to do. They make their best guess, but they're incorrect. Repeatedly and repeatedly. It's no surprise that children with poor listening skills frequently are thrown in jail or the school clown.

Be patient and positive with them. Don't be afraid of talking about your listening skills. The more your child is aware of the situation, the better they're willing to tackle the issue instead of becoming annoyed.

It's not all of it. I hope that you've gained new knowledge, new techniques and strategies assist your child in improving their communication and language abilities. If you've read this far, you'll be able to agree that having the ability to communicate and speak clearly are essential for a variety of reasons.

I would like you to keep in mind these things:

Be a good role model.

Use teachable moments.

Use praise and compliments LIBERALLY.

www.ingramcontent.com/pod-product-compliance
Lightning Source LLC
Chambersburg PA
CBHW050024130526
44590CB00042B/1898